Probiotics for Health

Probiotics for Health

100 Amazing and Unexpected Uses for Probiotics

Jo A. Panyko, BS, MNT
of PowerofProbiotics.com

Adams Media
New York   London   Toronto   Sydney   New Delhi

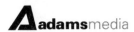

Adams Media
An Imprint of Simon & Schuster, Inc.
57 Littlefield Street
Avon, Massachusetts 02322

First Adams Media trade paperback edition AUGUST 2017

ADAMS MEDIA and colophon are trademarks of Simon and Schuster.

For information about special discounts for bulk purchases, please contact Simon & Schuster Special Sales at 1-866-506-1949 or business@simonandschuster.com.

The Simon & Schuster Speakers Bureau can bring authors to your live event. For more information or to book an event contact the Simon & Schuster Speakers Bureau at 1-866-248-3049 or visit our website at www.simonspeakers.com.

Manufactured in the United States of America

10 9 8 7 6 5 4 3 2 1

Library of Congress Cataloging-in-Publication Data has been applied for.

ISBN 978-1-5072-0427-6
ISBN 978-1-5072-0428-3 (ebook)

Many of the designations used by manufacturers and sellers to distinguish their products are claimed as trademarks. Where those designations appear in this book and Simon & Schuster, Inc., was aware of a trademark claim, the designations have been printed with initial capital letters.

The various uses of probiotics as health aids are based on tradition, scientific theories, or limited research. They often have not been thoroughly tested in humans, and safety and effectiveness have not yet been proven in clinical trials. Some of the conditions for which probiotics can be used as a treatment or remedy are potentially serious and should be evaluated by a qualified healthcare provider.

This book is intended as general information only, and should not be used to diagnose or treat any health condition. In light of the complex, individual, and specific nature of health problems, this book is not intended to replace professional medical advice. The ideas, procedures, and suggestions in this book are intended to supplement, not replace, the advice of a trained medical professional. Consult your physician before adopting any of the suggestions in this book, as well as about any condition that may require diagnosis or medical attention. The author and publisher disclaim any liability arising directly or indirectly from the use of this book.

Dedication

This book is dedicated to my brother, John A. Panyko, a generous soul and awesome attorney, who sometimes has the best advice for his little sister.

This book is also dedicated to you, its reader, who wonders if probiotics may help with your health problems or the problems of loved ones. May you find the answers you seek to lead you down a path to better health!

Acknowledgments

I want to acknowledge my family and friends, who provide love, encouragement, and support every day.

I especially want to thank my husband, Steve. Thanks for being the rock in my life to provide grounding, particularly when projects, events, and deadlines seem to be more difficult than they are. Your sense of humor, love, and positive outlook on life make the world a better place.

Lastly, I want to thank my children, Alison, Ellen, and Alex, for being my personal cheerleaders and bringing so much joy to my life.

CONTENTS

INTRODUCTION

If someone told you he had a product that could help resolve constipation and diarrhea, ward off infection, boost your immune system, assist your body in fighting off cancer, curb allergies, and even help you fight obesity, you would probably be pretty wary, but such a product does exist and you probably have it in your home at this very moment. This product is probiotics.

What exactly are probiotics? The World Health Organization defines *probiotics* as "Live microorganisms that, when administered in adequate amounts, confer a health benefit on the host." The term comes from the Latin preposition *pro* meaning "for" and the Greek word *biotikos* meaning "life." Probiotics are living microscopic creatures that you ingest to gain myriad health benefits—they are, in fact, beneficial microbes.

"Beneficial microbes" may seem like an oxymoron; after all, you no doubt have heard that microbes such as bacteria are bad, that they are the cause of illness and disease and must be eradicated from your home and living spaces if you want to stay healthy and germ-free. And while it is true that some microbes are bad for your body and do cause disease, this is not true for all microbes. In fact, in your body right now you have beneficial microorganisms that regulate your digestive system, immune system, and countless other body functions. These microbes are a necessary part of your body, but many of the things you do or consume can kill or injure them, leaving your body open to ailments.

Enter probiotics. These helpful microorgansims keep you functioning properly by helping you absorb important nutrients in your digestive tract, by reducing the presence of pathogens, and by regulating the removal of wastes out of your body. When you lose beneficial microbes—either through sickness or through certain medications like antibiotics or antifungals—it leaves your body vulnerable and then pathogenic forms of bacteria, viruses, and yeasts can take hold in your system causing everything from yeast infections and irritable bowl syndrome to eczema and hair loss.

There are now hundreds of known uses for probiotics that not only include digestive help but also benefits against many internal health conditions, from the common cold and asthma to certain forms of cancer. Probiotics can also help with your external health as well. They have been shown to help reduce the signs of aging, improve nails and hair, and even fight bad breath and acne. The benefits of probiotics can be felt throughout your entire body and mind.

In this book you will find 100 uses for probiotics to improve your health and well-being on the inside and the outside. You will learn how to take probiotics, which kind may be beneficial for your condition, and what the possible effects might be. You will discover that true health and beauty doesn't come from big pharma companies or in those expensive tubs of beauty creams and lotions; it comes (literally) from within your own body and promoting the health and numbers of your beneficial microbes. So let's get started on improving your health and your life!

PROBIOTICS AND THEIR MANY HEALTH BENEFITS

What Are Probiotics?

Probiotics are officially defined by the Joint Food and Agricultural Organization of the United Nations/World Health Organization Working Group as "Live microorganisms that, when administered in adequate amounts, confer a health benefit on the host." Basically, probiotics at this point in time are live bacteria and yeasts that provide health benefits to you if you take them in adequate quantities.

Probiotics are not drugs (in the United States), although super potent forms may be obtained through prescription. As such, they are not intended to treat or cure any diseases, mental or physical. Probiotics are a complement to a healthy way of life filled with nutritious food, adequate exercise, restorative sleep, beneficial social engagements, reduced exposure to toxins, and hydration with clean water.

Probiotics are part of your body's *microbiota*, your collection of microbes. The sum of the microbiota and its metabolic activities is called your *microbiome*. You will often see the word "microbiome" used to denote both the microbiota and its genetic and metabolic effects.

A Brief History of Probiotics

Microorganisms such as *Archaea* are believed by science to be the earliest life forms, with bacteria and yeasts, which are also microscopic organisms, not far behind. Although bacteria and yeast cells are much smaller than human cells, it may surprise you to know that your human cells have some basic processes in common with bacteria and yeasts.

Animals, including humans, have microbes inside them that benefit them in multiple ways. These microbes are in a loose sense like probiotics, but the definition of probiotics was established to designate those microbes that have been isolated, studied, tested in a laboratory dish and/or clinically in animals and/ or humans, and proven to have beneficial properties. In many cases their genetic fingerprints were sequenced for identification purposes and also to check for potentially harmful genetic components. The official term "probiotics" established specific criteria for scientific studies and probiotic supplements, foods, and drinks.

While most probiotics are found only in probiotic supplements, you can find some probiotics and/or other beneficial microbes on raw produce; in raw, fermented foods and beverages such as yogurt, sauerkraut, kimchi, some cheeses, kefir, kombucha, and kvass; and in probiotic-fortified processed foods such as some breads and chocolates. Specific types of microbes used as probiotics are outlined in the following "Overview of Probiotic Microbes" section. Probiotics and other beneficial microorganisms are best used preventively and with variety, so for optimum results, indulge in them daily.

The concept of probiotics is credited to Élie Metchnikoff, a Russian scientist born in the mid-1800s, whose work provided profound insights into immunology and microbes. He developed a theory about aging that over the years had been forgotten in mainstream medicine but is now embraced by many scientists: namely, that health is influenced by toxic bacteria in the gastrointestinal (GI) tract. He is said to have noticed that people who lived to be over 100 years old in the Balkan States and Russia drank sour milk, which we now call yogurt or kefir, every day. In fact, Bulgarian yogurt cultures even today are regarded as highly therapeutic.

The Special Benefits of Probiotics

How can something as small as a microscopic organism be so important for health? The reason is that there is not just one microbe, nor a handful; there are approximately 1 trillion microbes per gram of feces. Microbes within you are found on your mucous membranes, spanning from your mouth to your anus, from your nasal passages to your lungs, in your urinary tract, and even on your eyes. In fact, in your digestive tract alone, it is calculated that for every cell of yours that is human, there are an equal number of bacterial cells.

There are also microbes that live on your skin, and different types prefer to live in different niches of your skin. Microbiota, the collection of microorganisms, are well adapted to live in and on your body, and while they benefit from resources you provide, under normal circumstances you benefit much more from everything they do for you.

Inside your body bacterial and other microbial cells live in close contact with your own cells, and in healthy conditions the thing that separates them from you is a layer of mucus. Between that layer of mucus and the inside of you is a layer of skin-like cells one-cell thick. One thing you have to understand about your gastrointestinal (GI) tract is that although it resides within you, it is really connected to the outside world, from your lips to your anus, and the things that protect you from the outside world are the mucus; the skin-like layer of cells with immune, nervous, and endocrine cells below it; and the beneficial microbes. At least 70 percent of your immune system is in your GI tract!

The beneficial microbes, including probiotics, live with other microbes that are either benign, pathogenic (disease-causing), or opportunistic, meaning that they normally play nicely but can get out of control if given the opportunity. Actually, any microbe can cause you problems if it ends up in a place other than where it is supposed to be. Such a scenario can happen with intestinal permeability, commonly called *leaky gut*. Leaky gut happens when the layer of skin-like cells in your GI tract develops gaps in between the cells, allowing food particles, toxins, microbes, and other hazards to enter your bloodstream, if not stopped by the immune system.

Since mucus, the thin layer of cells, and your immune system are your only defenses against the outside world within your digestive tract, it is very beneficial to you to have helpful microbes protecting you from potentially pathogenic microbes. These beneficial microbes can produce acids or antimicrobial products called *bacteriocins*, which hinder or kill pathogens. They can also stand in solidarity to prevent pathogens from taking up residence, or displace them if they do.

But beneficial microbes such as probiotics do more than just protect you from pathogens inside and outside your body. Probiotics can have significant effects on your digestion and nutrient absorption. They can utilize food substances, such as soluble fibers, that otherwise would be useless to your nutrition. They can break down substances in foods that keep you from absorbing the micronutrients inside. They not only protect against the consequences of rogue molecules passing through a leaky gut, but they assist your intestinal cells in staying healthy to optimize nutrient absorption. In addition, some of the metabolic by-products of probiotics, such as short-chain fatty acids and vitamin production, are very nourishing to your GI tract.

Probiotics have direct and indirect effects on your immune system. They can help tip an imbalance in an immune response, such as in seasonal allergies, to a more balanced state. Probiotics have direct and indirect effects on your nervous and endocrine systems, too, and are part of your enteric nervous system. They can influence every system in your body. The amount of probiotics shown to be beneficial in research for various conditions differs based on the population and condition studied, so no blanket recommendations can be made.

Cautions

There are many benefits to probiotics, but there are also a few cautions to heed as well. First, if you are immune compromised (catheters, cancer treatments, HIV, trauma, and so on), please consult your physician to check if there are any contraindications for using probiotics. Second, if you never used probiotics or a particular type of probiotic before, and/or never ate much raw food or indulged in fermented foods and drinks (such as sauerkraut, kimchi, kefir, or kombucha), please proceed slowly with probiotic use. Although probiotics are tiny organisms, they can have very potent effects on your body.

As you progress with increasing dosages of probiotics internally, you may experience increased abdominal gas, upset digestion with diarrhea, headache, fever, muscle pain, brain fog, and/or anxiety. If the symptoms become too uncomfortable, decrease the dosage for a few days and try again. These symptoms are your body's way of telling you that things—such as a die-off of pathogens or an awakened intestinal reflex—are changing.

If you ever have shortness of breath, tightness in your throat, hives, or other symptoms of an allergic reaction, discontinue use immediately and seek medical help.

The side effects of probiotics as your body adapts to them are usually mild if you are generally healthy. Introduce probiotic foods, drinks, and supplements gradually and soon you will be reaping their benefits.

Overview of Probiotic Microbes

There are five main types of probiotics, each in its own classification called a *genus*. Within each genus there are multiple species, and within those species there are multiple strains. For example, *Lactobacillus* is a very common genus of probiotics.

Within that genus are numerous species, such as *rhamnosus*. The genus and species of a microbe are always italicized, making it easy to know that a microbe is involved. In a species such as *Lactobacillus rhamnosus* (often abbreviated *L. rhamnosus*), there are many strains. An example of the name of a strain is *L. rhamnosus* GR-1.

Here are the most common genera you will encounter:

- *Lactobacillus* is a common genus of probiotic, and at least thirteen different species are used as probiotics. *Lactobacillus* is a common resident of your GI tract and is also commonly found in the vagina. It is found on raw produce, in many fermented foods and drinks, and in probiotic supplements.
- *Bifidobacterium* is another common genus, with at least seven species used as probiotics. *Bifidobacterium* is a normal resident of your GI tract and is the dominant microbe in breast milk. Probiotic supplements and fermented milk products are the best sources of *Bifidobacterium*.
- *Streptococcus* has two species that are probiotics, *thermophilus* and *salivarius*. Most others act either neutrally or pathogenically in you. *Thermophilus* is found in yogurt. *Salivarius* is found in normal oral microbiota. Both species are found in supplements.
- *Bacillus* is an interesting genus because these microbes have the ability to form endospores, tough outer coatings, when conditions are not suitable for them to flourish. There are five species of probiotic *Bacillus*: *clausii, coagulans, indicus, licheniformis*, and *subtilis*. Not every species of *Bacillus* is probiotic. Some *Bacillus* species are usually pathogens. *Bacillus* may normally be found in the GI tract, but they generally do not take up residence for long and will pass through and be eliminated if not replenished. *Bacillus* are common food spoilage organisms and are also found in probiotic supplements and in soil, air, and water.
- Another genus of probiotic that passes through your GI tract is a yeast, *Saccharomyces*. There are two species used probiotically, *cerevisiae*, found in baker's and brewer's yeast, and *boulardii*, found in supplements.

There are other lesser-utilized probiotics, including some *Leuconostoc*, *Lactococcus*, and *Clostridium butyricum*, and *E. coli* Nissle, among others.

The world of probiotics and the gut microbiome is an exciting one that is impacting and will continue to impact how health and medicine are viewed. Read on to discover more about it!

1: CALMS REACTIONS TO FOODS

Different people react to foods differently. What may be nourishing to one person may be another person's poison. We don't normally think of foods as being poisonous because they usually are not deadly, but foods can be toxic to a person who is allergic, intolerant, or sensitive to them. The difference in toxicity may show in symptoms.

In a food allergy, there is an immediate immune reaction to the offensive food. Classic allergic symptoms such as tingling lips, burning/tightness in the mouth/throat, gastrointestinal upset, difficulty breathing, rashes, hives, and even anaphylaxis may be present. Although any food can cause an allergic reaction, the most common offenders are peanuts, tree nuts, dairy, fish, shellfish, eggs, soy, and wheat.

In a food intolerance, the body is not able to properly handle the food, but there is not an allergic reaction. A classic example is lactose intolerance. Please see the section on lactose intolerance for more information.

In a food sensitivity, the immune reaction is delayed, usually several hours to days after the exposure. Food sensitivities are the most difficult to determine since there is not an immediate reaction. These kinds of issues with foods can cause a wide range of physical and mental problems. An elimination diet followed by reintroduction is one of the best ways to determine a food sensitivity.

Food allergies and sensitivities both involve the immune system, albeit in different ways. Many types of probiotics can help modulate the immune system, and they can calm these conditions, not only via immune regulation, but also through prevention of intestinal permeability, improved intestinal motility, and communication with your genes.

2: LESSENS SEASONAL ALLERGY REACTIONS

Seasonal respiratory allergies can cause itchy, watery eyes, scratchy throat, and an annoying runny, stuffy nose. Often called *hay fever*, seasonal respiratory allergies are your body's response to otherwise innocuous substances such as pollen, outdoor mold spores, dust, and animal dander. These substances are *allergens*. Some allergens are only present in large quantities in the spring and fall. Others are present throughout the year. You might have allergies to different allergens that could leave you suffering year-round.

The reason for your suffering is an overreaction by your body to the allergens. Your body detects these allergens and mounts a massive immune response attack against them, including the release of histamine and other chemicals in a futile attempt to protect you. Many times there is a threshold at which you can no longer tolerate your total allergen load, and that is when symptoms balloon. Aside from monitoring allergen counts and avoiding allergens as much as possible (also vacuuming frequently, reducing carpeting, washing bedding frequently, and so on), did you know that there are other treatment options besides allergy shots and antihistamines?

Oral probiotics are helpful because 70–80 percent of your immune system is in your gastrointestinal tract, so ingesting various forms of probiotics can help balance your immune system from the inside out. Probiotics species in the *Bifidobacterium* and *Lactobacillus* genera as well as some *Bacillus* have shown efficacy in reducing seasonal allergic symptoms. Probiotics work best preventively, so take them year-round.

In addition to diet and lifestyle modifications, probiotics help get to the root of the problem and calm down the response of the immune system to seasonal allergens.

3: IMPROVES ANEMIA

Are you feeling run down? Getting sick frequently? You could have a case of common iron-deficiency anemia. Your body needs small amounts of iron, carried in hemoglobin in red blood cells in your blood, to carry oxygen to tissues for energy production and to act as a catalyst in various reactions in the body.

Iron-deficiency anemia can be caused by blood loss (menstruation, ulcers, hemorrhoids, and colon cancer, among others); inability to meet the body's needs (pregnancy, childbirth, recovery from injury, and cancers); and increased destruction of red blood cells (from inherited conditions such as sickle cell anemia and thalassemia, or toxins such as venom, drugs, or trauma).

Sometimes iron absorption from foods is not enough for your needs, and in the case of diagnosed iron-deficiency anemia, iron supplements may be necessary to bring your body's stores of iron to normal levels. Probiotics can help your body better absorb iron from foods so that you get adequate amounts for your everyday needs, and they can help you absorb iron from supplements too.

One of the ways probiotics help is by producing acids that help keep iron in a soluble form. *Lactobacillus*, *Streptococcus thermophilus*, *Bifidobacterium*, *Lactococcus*, and some *Bacillus* can do that. Another way is by breaking down antinutrients in foods such as phytates, which bind iron in unusable forms, so that the iron becomes available. Yet other ways probiotics help with your body's iron needs is by maintaining the gastrointestinal (GI) barrier and combating ulcer development to prevent iron losses through blood, and by protecting GI mucus and cells that hold and release iron in the GI tract.

Maintaining adequate levels of iron in the body is important for health, and probiotics can help!

4: SOOTHES ACHY JOINTS

Do you ever feel like the Tin Man from *The Wizard of Oz* movie? Having osteoarthritis can feel like you need lubrication in your joints to get you moving. Osteoarthritis (OA) is a degenerative joint disease in which the cartilage in a joint becomes damaged, joint movement is restricted, and pain ensues. The most common joints affected are the knees and hips, and it is not uncommon to experience OA in multiple joints.

Many people believe that OA is a normal wear-and-tear condition and that getting it is inevitable as you age. Indeed, statistics in the UK show that 33 percent of people forty-five years old and older and 49 percent of women and 42 percent of men aged seventy-five years and over have sought medical treatment for the disease.

However, even though there may be some genetic links, experiencing disabling osteoarthritis is not inevitable as you age. Being overweight is a major risk factor for OA development, mainly because your joints were not meant to move excessive amounts of weight, but also because carrying extra weight increases your body's inflammatory state. That is why anti-inflammatory medications, such as ibuprofen, are commonly prescribed for OA.

Taking anti-inflammatory medications can help with inflammation and pain, but they are not addressing some of the root causes of why OA happened in the first place. Weight loss, smoking cessation, eating a diet focused on vegetables, taking popular supplements such as glucosamine and chondroitin (among others), and taking probiotics may soothe your achy joints. Caring for your gut health with a variety of probiotics can help OA by reducing the inflammatory chemicals, which attack collagen in the joints and contribute to inflammation and pain, produced by pathogens and problems in your gut.

5: LOWERS RHEUMATOID ARTHRITIS ACTIVITY

Do you have joint pain with swelling and stiffness, and possibly redness, especially that which lasts longer than a half-hour in the mornings? These could be symptoms of rheumatoid arthritis.

Rheumatoid arthritis (RA) is an autoimmune form of arthritis that attacks the lining of your joints. This means that your body mistakenly attacks its own tissues due to immune system dysregulation. RA typically begins in the joints of the feet or fingers, but it can affect any joints and is likely to progress if no action is taken. Repeated episodes of joint inflammation can result in damage to joints and instability in joints, with deformities being common. This repeated inflammation can lead to great disability.

Conventional treatment of RA involves painkillers, anti-inflammatory drugs, disease-modifying antirheumatic drugs (which target inflammatory molecules), and steroids to suppress the autoimmune attack. Genetics may play a role in RA, but it is not the cause. Cold, damp weather may aggravate the condition, but it is not the cause either. As with most autoimmune diseases, it takes a trigger to switch on the autoimmunity. The trigger could be something such as diet, lifestyle, environmental toxins, or stress. The keys to preventing or managing RA are to lessen repeated triggers and keep the antioxidant and immune systems balanced so that inflammation is minimized.

Since 70–80 percent of your immune system is in your gastrointestinal tract, oral probiotics offer a nontoxic way to balance it. Research into specific probiotic strains and RA is in its infancy, but trials with *Lactobacillus casei*, *Lactobacillus acidophilus*, *Lactobacillus salivarius*, and *Bifidobacterium bifidum* have shown promise in significantly decreasing the RA disease-activity scores of participants.

6: IMPROVES ASTHMA

Asthma is a chronic inflammatory immune disorder that affects the airway passages of susceptible children and adults. Symptoms can include wheezing, chest tightness, coughing, and difficulty breathing. Asthma sufferers typically also have allergies.

The most common prescribed medications to treat asthma are steroids to suppress inflammation, bronchodilators to open airways, and medications to block an allergic response. Peak flow meters are often used as a simple test of lung function to alert asthma suffers of the status of their breathing capacity.

Many studies suggest that the best time to prevent asthma is in infancy, when a child's immune system is undergoing rapid maturation. Therefore, most studies involving probiotics in the management or prevention of asthma are conducted on infants and young children. Results show that children with a more diverse bacterial community are less likely to develop asthma. Chewable tablets or oral drops of probiotics, and beneficial microbes from raw produce, fermented foods and drinks, and supplements, can help with immune system development and microbial diversity in young children.

The microbial balance in airways also is disrupted in people with asthma compared to those without. Studies with probiotics for asthma in adults are limited, but recent treatments including probiotic formulas containing *Bifidobacterium breve* or *Clostridium butyricum* were shown to improve asthma.

RELIEF MAY START IN THE GUT

Asthma is a complicated disease, with many triggers and unspecified causes, but it is known that asthma is an immune disorder. Since 70–80 percent of your immune system is in your intestines, and since immune molecules can travel from the gastrointestinal tract to sites all over the body, including the airways, balancing the microbiota there with the help of targeted probiotics to counteract the dysbiosis present may provide asthma symptom relief.

7: SHOWS PROMISE FOR HELPING AUTISM

Autism is a wide-spectrum developmental disorder triggered in early childhood and characterized by repetitive behaviors and difficulties in social interactions and communication. There is no recognized cure. The exact trigger is unknown, but some interplay between genetics and environmental factors is suspected. One theory that is gaining momentum is that an imbalance in gastrointestinal (GI) microbes sets the stage for autism to develop.

An imbalance in the GI microbiota has the potential to directly affect the digestive system, immune system, brain/nervous system, and endocrine system, and inflammatory molecules from the GI tract can travel throughout the body to other systems. Since children's immune systems develop over time after birth, any assault to the digestive, immune, nervous, or endocrine systems via an imbalance in GI microbiota has the potential to affect development.

The majority of children with autism have severe GI disorders such as abdominal pain, diarrhea, constipation, or irritable bowel disease. These disorders in adults and children without autism have been linked to gut microbiota disruptions.

Studies show that children with autism also have less bacterial diversity in their GI tracts, and in general, less diversity is associated with reduced health. To explore the gut microbiota–autism connection, recent trials with probiotics and fecal transplants in autistic children and in animals with induced autistic symptoms have shown great promise by improving the microbial diversity, digestive health, and behavioral symptoms in those subjects.

RESEARCH IT

Several prominent doctors, including Dr. Natasha Campbell-McBride, the author of *Gut and Psychology Syndrome* and creator of the GAPS diet, focus on the status of the GI tract for prevention and in their treatments of autism and other disorders. More information about her and her GAPS diet can be found at www.doctor-natasha.com.

8: REDUCES VAGINAL INFLAMMATION

Aerobic vaginitis (AV) is a form of vaginal inflammation that is often confused with or may be combined with other forms of vaginal infections. It is important to distinguish which bacteria are causing the infection so that appropriate medications or treatments can be prescribed. Severe forms of the infection may be called desquamative inflammatory vaginitis. AV shares some symptoms of other vaginal infections, namely itching or burning, painful intercourse, unusual yellow discharge, and inflammation.

A healthy vagina is commonly populated by various species of anaerobic (not oxygen dependent) bacteria, such as *Lactobacillus*. In AV, pathogenic species of bacteria that require oxygen (aerobic) or can tolerate oxygen take up residence. Some of these bacteria may be from feces or the environment. These aerobic bacteria overwhelm the resident beneficial bacteria and cause an infection. The infection increases immune cells in the vagina, and yet decreases the ability of those immune cells to do their jobs.

As you might imagine, probiotic *Lactobacillus* species, taken preventively internally or inserted vaginally during and after symptoms, can help control the populations of bacteria that cause AV both in the gastrointestinal tract as well as the vagina. They do this by lowering the pH of the environment, crowding out pathogens, preventing pathogenic bacteria from adhering to tissues, causing the harmful bacteria to disengage from tissues, and producing antimicrobial substances to disable/kill the pathogens.

Remember, if you suspect you have aerobic vaginitis or any other kind of vaginal infection based on your symptoms, even if you are using probiotics, please see a healthcare professional for an accurate diagnosis.

DON'T SELF-DIAGNOSE

Aerobic vaginitis can be a serious infection. If you suspect you have AV, please see a healthcare professional for proper diagnosis. Only a healthcare professional can diagnose aerobic vaginitis, so please do not try to self-diagnose.

9: COMBATS BACTERIAL VAGINOSIS

Bacterial vaginosis (BV) is a common form of vaginal infection that is often considered a stealth infection, meaning you can have it and not know it. If symptoms are present, they usually involve itchiness and a vaginal discharge with a strong, fishy odor. The odor can help distinguish BV from other forms of vaginitis, but the infection can only be correctly diagnosed by a healthcare professional.

BV disrupts the normal microbial environment in the vagina, which can increase the risk of HIV transmission and other sexually transmitted diseases (STDs). This disruption can also increase the risk of serious infections with intrauterine devices (IUDs) or from surgical procedures, and the infection can spread to the uterus and fallopian tubes resulting in serious complications. Significantly, BV in pregnant mothers increases the risks of premature delivery and babies born with low birth weight.

The exact cause of BV is not known, but introduction of any outside influences (multiple partners, douching, IUDs) are risk factors. The end result in BV is a disruption in the healthy balance of microbes in the vagina. Conventional treatments involve the use of antibiotics to attempt to kill the pathogenic bacteria. Typically multiple courses of antibiotics are necessary, and there are high relapse rates.

Another way to combat BV is through the consistent use of probiotics, allowing the beneficial bacteria to reduce the number and impact of the pathogenic bacteria. Many different species of probiotics have shown efficacy, but the most well-known used acutely are *Lactobacillus rhamnosus* GR-1 and *Lactobacillus reuteri* RC-14.

CAUTION: SERIOUS INFECTION

Bacterial vaginosis can be a serious infection with the potential to affect other organs and the health of a developing fetus. If you suspect you have BV, please see a healthcare professional for proper diagnosis.

10: REDUCES RISKS ASSOCIATED WITH BURN INJURY

Burn injury is the fourth-leading cause of injury from trauma, according to the World Health Organization. It is also a major cause of unintentional child injury death and accounts for a portion of military-related accidents. Because of the severity of the injuries associated with burns, new developments to improve survival and quality of life for survivors are necessary.

Patients with large total body-surface-area burns and third-degree burns, particularly, are at risk of serious infections. Extensive burn injuries usually require grafting and extended hospital stay, but infection can delay the procedures.

Burn injury infection following serious burns occurs frequently due to immune suppression, wound microbial colonization, and development of treatment-resistant microbes due to the length of antibiotic treatment required. There is also a high risk of graft failure in burn injury patients.

Research into the use of probiotics, both topically and taken orally, for burn injury patients is in progress. Initial results are encouraging, with patients provided an oral mix of *Lactobacillus*, *Bifidobacterium*, and *Streptococcus* bacteria having more successful graft takes. In mice with burn injury, topical application of *Lactobacillus plantarum* reduced the translocation of pathogens to internal organs and suppressed the formation of infection-related chemicals. Therefore, probiotics may reduce risks associated with burn injury.

ACT QUICKLY WHEN BURNS OCCUR

Prevention is the best way to prevent burn injuries, particularly with children. If you or someone you know has been badly burned, please seek emergency treatment immediately. Doing so can reduce the chances of infection and possible death, and can also reduce the chances of scarring and disfigurement.

11: ADDS TO BREAST CANCER PREVENTION ARSENAL

Breast cancer can affect men as well as women. While there are many types of breast cancers and numerous treatments, there are common preventative actions that everyone can take.

The risk factors for breast cancer are many, and you do not have control over some of them, like your age or race. However, you do have control over many other risk factors, such as alcohol use, sex hormone levels, body weight, intake of vegetables and fruits, and level of physical activity.

One area of breast cancer research that is expanding is the use of probiotics for prevention or concurrent treatment. Probiotics can help protect against some risk factors, like toxic alcohol by-products, as well as help to balance sex hormones. One of the ways they do this is through protection of the liver. When the liver is protected from damaging molecules caused by unbalanced microbiota in the gastrointestinal tract, it can function more efficiently to break down toxic products and excess hormones.

Another way probiotics can help is by assisting with regularity. Bowel movements rid the body of excess hormones, toxins, and waste products. Probiotics also can help you use many of the anticancer plant compounds in vegetables and fruits, maintain a healthy body weight, and increase your level of activity by affecting your moods, aches and pains, and endurance.

Adding probiotics to your arsenal of breast cancer prevention interventions is an easy thing to do!

12: MAY HELP IN COLON CANCER PREVENTION

There is blood in your stool and you immediately think you have colon cancer, but do you? Blood in the stool can also be caused by ulcers or polyps, but the only way to know for sure is to have your situation diagnosed by a healthcare professional.

Other signs of colon cancer are a change in consistency and frequency of bowel movements, persistent abdominal cramps, a feeling of incomplete evacuation of the bowels, weakness and fatigue, and unexplained weight loss. What you may not know, however, is that early in the development of colon cancer you may not have any discernable symptoms. That is why prevention and routine screenings are so important.

While there is no agreed cause of colon cancer, what can be agreed upon is that aberrant mutations in colon cells lead to errors in DNA. These errors, if not caught by the immune system, can lead to uncontrolled cell division with the mutations intact, resulting in tumors.

Some risk factors for colon cancer are older age, history of polyps, inflammatory intestinal disorders, sedentary lifestyle, and diet choices among others. Probiotics can help in the prevention of colon cancer in many ways. One way is that they help maintain consistent elimination patterns, especially as you age, so that the stool does not sit in the colon for an extended period of time. Another way is that they can reduce inflammation in the colon (thereby reducing the chances of aberrant DNA mistakes), by reducing pathogens, preserving intestinal integrity, and soothing inflammation with anti-inflammatory effects.

Combining different probiotics from a variety of sources daily, along with a diet focused on lean proteins, healthy fats, moderate amounts of fruits and plenty of colorful vegetables, as well as a lifestyle focused on movement, may be the best ways to prevent common causes of colon cancer.

13: OFFERS HELP IN LIVER CANCER PREVENTION

Liver cancer is disabling to the body because your liver is critical to your survival. It is your main internal detoxification organ. It also performs numerous unique functions such as protein assemblage, controlling amounts of nutrients in the blood, bile synthesis, and many others.

The most common type of liver cancer, and the second most deadly cancer in the world, is hepatocellular carcinoma (HCC). Some risk factors for HCC are any condition that impairs liver function, such as alcoholism, obesity, hepatitis B or C, nonalcoholic fatty liver disease, and cirrhosis.

Many people do not realize that the health of their gastrointestinal (GI) tract influences the health of their liver. If the GI tract is functioning normally and has balanced microbiota, then excess hormones and other waste products are properly eliminated rather than recirculated back to the liver. Also, production of toxins by pathogenic microbes, which can enter the portal vein to the liver, are reduced, and liver-damaging inflammatory chemicals are reduced. All of these functions ease the burden of an overloaded liver so it can function optimally.

Additionally, keeping the immune system balanced in the GI tract with beneficial microbes such as probiotics allows the immune system to deal with its everyday functions of surveillance and cleanup to reduce aberrant DNA mutations and to further reduce stress on the liver.

Studies in rodents show that many different types of probiotics can slow the progression of liver cancer tumor progression. Until human studies are performed to reveal the strains and dosages of probiotics for HCC prevention and treatment, the best thing to do to reduce your risk of HCC is to treat your liver kindly by reducing your risk factors and keeping your GI tract healthy with nutritious foods and probiotics.

14: REDUCES CARDIOVASCULAR DISEASE RISKS

Cardiovascular disease occurs in the heart and/or blood vessels and manifests as heart attacks, stroke, hypertension (elevated blood pressure), peripheral artery disease, rheumatic and congenital heart diseases, and heart failure. It is the number one cause of death in the world, causing nearly one-third of all deaths.

Although there may be a minor influence of genetics, the major causes of cardiovascular disease are factors within your control: tobacco use, lack of physical exercise, an unhealthy diet, and overindulgence in alcohol. One thing that all of these causes have in common is that they increase inflammation and oxidative stress in the body. Another thing is that they contribute to disruption in the oral and gut microbiota.

In microbiota disruption, dominant nonprobiotic microbes in the gut produce toxins that may be carried throughout the body to affect organs and tissues, such as the heart and its blood vessels. Additionally, nonprobiotic microbes are able to break down substances in some foods to produce trimethylamines, which are associated with atherosclerosis (plaque buildup in arteries) and cardiac events.

Taking a variety of probiotics, in addition to reducing your other risk factors, helps prevent an imbalance in your oral and gut microbiota. Without a major imbalance, numbers of non-probiotic, nonbeneficial bacteria and yeasts will be low and the toxic substances they produce or contribute to will be minimized, thereby reducing your cardiovascular disease risks.

REDUCE HEART DISEASE RISKS

You can reduce your chances or the severity of cardiovascular disease by working on the risk factors you can control. For example, don't use tobacco, get movement in your day, eat nutritious foods, limit alcohol intake, and take probiotics. Nutritious foods, in particular, will not only nourish you, but they will nourish the beneficial microbes in your digestive tract.

15: HELPS TO BALANCE CHOLESTEROL

Do you know your cholesterol numbers? Many doctors and patients are fixated on lowering them, which is why statin drugs are popularly prescribed. While there is debate over the relevance of general cholesterol numbers in cardiovascular disease, in the spirit of cholesterol reduction, there are dietary and lifestyle things you can do. As an added benefit, these things do not have side effects, such as the muscle aches/weakness, headaches and other neurological symptoms, and numerous gastrointestinal complications that often accompany statin usage.

Cholesterol is a vital substance for you, so levels that are too low are not healthy. Although people worry about cholesterol levels in foods, for most people cholesterol is primarily manufactured in their livers from simple carbohydrates, trans fats, and saturated fats. Reducing your intake of the first two and eating saturated fats from animals fed their native diets, without antibiotics or hormones, can help improve cholesterol levels.

Probiotics can also help maintain healthy cholesterol levels, mainly through their impact on bile. Cholesterol is an ingredient in bile, which is formed in the liver, stored in the gallbladder, and released into the small intestine to help solubilize dietary fats. Most bile is reabsorbed and recirculated back to the liver several times. Probiotics can help interrupt the reabsorption, allowing the bile to be excreted as waste in feces and forcing the formation of new bile from cholesterol. They also reduce other factors that contribute to high cholesterol.

Some probiotic supplements on the market contain a strain of *Lactobacillus reuteri* that research has shown can reduce cholesterol levels. While probiotics alone may not reduce cholesterol as drastically as statin drugs, combining them with nutritious foods and an active lifestyle can achieve balanced cholesterol levels in most people with none of the side effects of statins.

CAUTION WITH MEDICATIONS

Do not stop taking any prescription without consulting your doctor. Incorporating lifestyle changes may require an adjustment to your statin dose.

16: MAY REDUCE DURATION AND SEVERITY OF COLDS

Ah, the misery: the stuffy, runny nose with sneezing; the sore, scratchy throat and cough; and the achiness and fatigue making you want to go back to bed. On average, according to the US Centers for Disease Control and Prevention, adults have an average of two to three colds per year, and children suffer from more. Recovery is typically within seven to ten days, but in people with compromised immune systems or respiratory conditions, the cold can progress into something more serious.

Colds are caused by viruses, not bacteria, so antibiotics cannot help resolve colds. Your body's immune system protects you against invaders such as cold viruses, but sometimes the immune system is overwhelmed or is not supported with proper nutrition and lifestyle.

There are simple ways to prevent getting a cold, such as washing your hands frequently and thoroughly with plain soap and water, keeping your dirty hands away from your face, and avoiding those who are sick. Sometimes it is not possible to do these things, and that is when you really have to rely on a strong and balanced immune system to keep you healthy.

A variety of probiotics can help with that. One of the major actions of probiotics is modulating the immune system, so that when you need immediate responders for an invader like a cold, the troops are ready and can go in with the correct and proper amount of ammunition and scale back their attack as needed to prevent further injury. Probiotics may reduce the duration and severity of colds, and using them prophylactically for all of their numerous benefits may help prevent you from succumbing to colds in the first place.

17: SOOTHES COLIC

Endless crying or wailing, sleepless nights both for baby and parents, and feelings of helplessness are common in colic. If your baby has colic, you are not alone. It is estimated that up to 25 percent of infants suffer from colic.

Sometimes the underlying cause is easy to discern, such as when the breastfeeding mother eliminates milk from her diet, or when the formula-fed baby is switched off milk-based formula. Other times the causes are not obvious. Breastfeeding mothers may be advised to eliminate cruciferous vegetables such as broccoli, cabbage, and cauliflower, as well as garlic and onions or spicy foods, to prevent the carryover of these foods into breast milk. However, indiscriminately eliminating such foods can have health consequences to the mother and to the nutrition content of her breast milk.

Babies with colic are frequently given simethicone drops, a medication to reduce gas formation in the baby's digestive tract. Since colic appears to be a problem in the digestive system, probiotics may help. Indeed, research shows that colicky babies have less diversity in their gastrointestinal (GI) microbiota, and it is well-known in the probiotics world that less diversity in the GI tract usually equates to a less healthy body. Research also shows that different species of probiotics in the *Lactobacillus* and *Bifidobacterium* genera as well as *Streptococcus thermophilus* can soothe the symptoms of colic and in some cases resolve the issue.

MOTHER AND BABY CAN BENEFIT

Since babies need a variety of beneficial microbes in their system for normal, healthy development and to possibly avoid future health conditions, probiotics taken by the breastfeeding mother as well as probiotics given in drop form to babies may ease the misery of colic for baby and parents. Please consult a healthcare professional if you have any concerns about using probiotics with yourself or your baby.

18: RELIEVES CONSTIPATION

Do you strain with infrequent bowel movements? Do the feces look like separate hard lumps or like bunches of hard lumps stuck together, or are they pencil-thin? You may have constipation. The Bristol stool chart (BSC) was developed by two doctors as a way to differentiate between states of constipation, normal elimination, a state of lacking fiber, and states of inflammation. Stools are supposed to be long and sausage-like, with few or no cracks in the surface.

The bad news about constipation is that there can be many causes, from simple causes like dehydration and lack of fiber to complicated structural causes or disease. While constipation may seem to be only a nuisance that causes uncomfortable symptoms such as abdominal bloating or pain, the truth is that constipation increases the risks of several diseases.

The reason constipation is linked to disease is that it allows undigested food and bodily wastes to sit in the colon, putrefy, and dry out. As feces dry out, water from the feces is reabsorbed back into the body, and along with it toxins. Additionally, microbes that like those conditions can multiply, releasing their toxic products that are then absorbed into your bloodstream.

Thankfully, most causes of constipation can be improved with dietary and lifestyle interventions. One of those interventions may be probiotics. Probiotics of many kinds can help with constipation because they can keep the digestive contents moving along through different mechanisms such as short-chain fatty acid production, influences on the nerves of the digestive tract, electrolyte balance, pathogen control, and others. Think of probiotics as an addition to other dietary and lifestyle interventions to relieve constipation and return your digestive system to its normal functions.

TO MAKE A DISH THAT CAN HELP WITH CONSTIPATION

Top your favorite salad loaded with greens, numerous vegetables, and avocado with one-quarter cup of raw sauerkraut instead of a questionable bottled salad dressing to restore health to your digestive tract and to get wastes moving.

19: HELPS WITH COMPLICATIONS OF CYSTIC FIBROSIS

Cystic fibrosis (CF) is a heritable genetic disorder that affects mucus-, sweat-, and digestive-juice-producing cells. As a result, thick mucus builds up, inhibiting the function of the lungs, pancreas, liver, intestines, and other organs. People with CF are at increased risk of lung infections and digestive system problems.

Mucus buildup in the lungs allows the balance of bacteria to become distorted and infections with pathogens to develop. Mucus accumulation in the pancreas prevents the release of digestive enzymes into the small intestine, thus impairing digestion and absorption. Mucus in the liver and bile ducts can cause liver disease as well as block bile from flowing into the small intestine. Without sufficient bile, not only is digestion and absorption reduced, but the balance of bacteria in the intestines becomes skewed. This results in an imbalance in gut microbiota that can lead to problems in every body system.

Probiotics can help with some of the complications of CF. For example, because of the increased risk of infections, people with CF are often prescribed antibiotics. Antibiotics kill pathogenic bacteria, but also kill the beneficial ones, too, causing an imbalance in microbes in the lungs and digestive tract and impaired functioning. Probiotics can help restore a balanced microbiota.

While balancing the microbiota, probiotics can also help with digestion, nutrient absorption, and systemic inflammation by producing short-chain fatty acids, keeping the intestinal cell layer intact to prevent rogue molecules from entering the bloodstream, regulating the motions of the intestines for proper elimination, and balancing the immune system.

NOT ONE PROBIOTIC FOR EVERYONE

CF affects people differently and research into probiotics and CF is in its infancy. One particular probiotic genus or strain hasn't been found to be more efficacious than any other. Speak to your healthcare professionals and see if a trial of a well-studied strain(s) may be right for you.

20: OFFERS HELP FOR DIABETES

Diabetes is a chronic disease characterized by the inability of the pancreas to produce insulin or by the inability of the body to properly use the insulin it produces. There are three main types of diabetes. Type 1 diabetes is an autoimmune condition in which the body's own cells attack pancreatic insulin-producing cells. Type 2 diabetes is the most prevalent type, believed to be mainly caused by dietary and lifestyle factors. Gestational diabetes occurs during pregnancy.

What all three types have in common is dysregulation of blood glucose. Elevated blood glucose is extremely damaging to the body, causing oxidative stress and inflammatory harms such as neuropathy (with amputation risk), blindness, kidney failure, and cardiovascular disease.

When you eat, your pancreas releases insulin to shuttle blood glucose from digested food to the bloodstream and into cells for energy production or for storage in the form of glycogen or fat. Too much fat in the body or too little exercise inhibits this process. Ingestion of too many carbohydrates, in particular, causes repeated spikes in blood glucose with necessary insulin release (or injection). Too much insulin in the blood for any reason leads to insulin resistance, the inability of cells to use available insulin. This can happen in all three forms of diabetes.

Simple measures, such as including a variety of probiotics and beneficial microbes, may help with prevention or management of all three types of diabetes. One of the ways probiotics can help is through energy regulation. They can use the carbohydrates you eat, especially the complex ones, and turn them into short-chain fatty acids (SCFA). SCFA influence the immune system to reduce oxidative stress and inflammation, decrease serum glucose, and improve insulin resistance.

CHECK YOUR BLOOD SUGAR LEVELS

Probiotics and other beneficial microbes may reduce your need for medications or the dosages of medications. Always monitor your blood sugar levels and report any concerns to your doctor.

21: REGULATES DIARRHEA

Diarrhea not only makes you feel unwell on the inside, but it can be embarrassing and cause skin irritation from the burning stools and odorous gas. Taking antidiarrheal medications is not addressing the cause(s). If you have diarrhea, your digestive system is not working well. Food is passing through you too quickly.

The Bristol stool chart (BSC) was developed by two doctors as a way to differentiate between states of constipation, normal elimination, a state of lacking fiber, and states of inflammation. Stools are supposed to be long and sausage-like, with few or no cracks in the surface. In diarrhea, stools are softer than normal, and may be very watery.

There are many types of diarrhea, such as acute, known-virus-related, food-pathogen-related, *C. difficile*-related, cholera, traveler's, enteral-nutrition-related, and antibiotic-associated. In each of these types, the causes may be different, but the results are the same.

When you eat, food is supposed to travel through the digestive system in about twenty-four hours, depending on what you eat and drink. When food remains reach the colon, excess water and nutrients are supposed to be absorbed. In diarrhea, the transit time from start to finish is reduced. Probiotics can help regulate the transit time to reduce diarrhea.

MANY PROBIOTICS

Although the strains of probiotics that have shown the best efficacy for diarrhea differ based on the type of diarrhea, taking any probiotic may help with the cause(s). By reducing pathogens, regulating contractions of the intestines, reducing oxidative stress and inflammation, increasing digestion and absorption, and balancing electrolytes, the end result of probiotic intervention is improvement in diarrhea. Please see your doctor if diarrhea persists.

22: BOOSTS IMMUNITY AGAINST FLU

Ugh, the coughing, sneezing, runny nose, spells of burning up followed by spells of freezing, pounding head, and an achy feeling that someone just beat you to a pulp...yes, my friend, you have the flu.

Flu is short for influenza, an upper respiratory viral infection. The main problem for you, and the main advantage for the survival of influenza viruses, is that there are many variations that can cause illness. Flu shots are based on virus strains that are anticipated to be widespread. Sometimes those assumptions are correct and other times they are not. This section will show you one overlooked way to fortify your body to best avoid becoming sick with the flu at all, or how to recover if you do succumb.

Viruses like the flu need you to survive, so they infect your cells. Once inside the safe harbor, they divide like there is no tomorrow. It isn't long before your immune system catches on to what is happening and mounts its attack.

You may have heard that taking vitamin C or zinc is helpful, preventively or during sickness. This is because vitamin C and zinc improve the functioning of cells of your innate immunity, your first line of defense against pathogens like the flu. They also are involved in the generation of and protection against the inflammatory response caused by the battle with the flu.

One overlooked mechanism that supports your innate immunity is gut health, specifically the role probiotics play. Probiotics keep your gut microbiota, inflammation, and immune system balanced preventively, as well as acutely when you are sick, so that no matter which flu strain comes along, your immune system is ready.

23: MINIMIZES FOOD POISONING AMBUSH

Food poisoning is really a misnomer, because it is not the food itself that is making you sick, but rather the pathogens in it. In most cases, pathogenic bacteria such as *Salmonella* or *Clostridium* are to blame. These pathogens can multiply on the inside and/or outside of food, even if the food is frozen for a while. If their numbers are high enough when you eat the food, you get sick.

Food pathogens are able to make you so sick because they are tenacious; they either infect your own cells or resort to a protective spore form when threatened. Their toxins are particularly potent and destructive, so keeping their numbers very low within you is important to avoid food poisoning.

One way to keep their numbers low is to keep your digestive tract balanced with beneficial microbes such as probiotics. If your system is balanced, it is better able to handle an assault because the intruders cannot gain access to you, and the probiotics and other beneficial microbes are there to fight on your behalf. If, however, your gut is already tipped in favor of pathogens, chances are that eating a tainted food is going to affect you more severely. It is possible that by taking a larger dose than normal of probiotics that you can mitigate the damage done and shorten the recovery time.

DEAL WITH THE INTRUDERS

Another way probiotics can help you avoid or deal with food poisoning is by balancing your immune system. When you have food poisoning, your innate immune molecules respond. They are designed to be the first line of immune defense and are trained to deal with intruders. Probiotics help your immune system do a proper job and help you be prepared for an ambush by food poisoning!

24: MANAGES DIGESTIVE HEALTH IN FOOD TUBE FEEDING

Food tube feeding, or enteral nutrition, is a necessity in the lives of many people. Whether it is a short-term measure or lifelong requirement, food tube feeding can provide nutrition directly to the digestive tract when a person has trouble chewing or swallowing, or has trouble with proper functioning of his or her digestive tract.

While food tube feeding provides nutrition necessary for survival, it is not without complications. Gastrointestinal (GI) complications such as constipation, bloating, diarrhea, malabsorption of nutrients, nausea, vomiting, electrolyte imbalances, dehydration, blood sugar fluctuations, and nutrient deficiencies may occur. Part of the reason for these complications is that food tube nutrition is usually in a liquid form. Without solid food, the GI tract does not get the proper signals to regulate peristalsis, the movement of food along the GI tract.

Also, a liquid diet, while providing the basic nutrients necessary for survival, cannot provide the thousands of phytochemicals and other nutrients from whole, real foods, unless supplemented with specially formulated puréed foods given as a bolus. Puréed foods may not be appropriate in some circumstances, so please check with a physician first.

Since it is not in solid form, food tube feeding usually does not contain beneficial microbes such as those found on raw foods, in fermented foods, or in probiotic supplements, nor substantial fiber. The lack of such microbes and fiber does not support a healthy gut microbiota. Gut microbiota, balanced by probiotics, can reduce the complications found during enteral feeding, as the sections in this book on constipation, diarrhea, and so on explain.

CONSULT YOUR PHYSICIAN FIRST

Care must be taken with probiotics anytime a person is being serviced by a tube due to the possibility of inadvertent microbial infection. While probiotics may alleviate some of the GI discomforts in food tube feeding, please check with a qualified physician before using them.

25: LESSENS RISK OF GALLSTONES

Gallstones are hard deposits in your gallbladder. If too many are present or they cause symptoms of possible bile duct obstruction, such as sudden onset of increasing pain just under your ribs or shoulder blades, or jaundice or high fever, emergency surgery may be necessary.

Your gallbladder is a small, pear-shaped organ connected to your liver and small intestine via bile ducts. Its purpose is to store excess bile from the liver so that adequate stores are available to help digest fats and act as signaling molecules in the gastrointestinal tract. The presence of fats in your small intestine signals a hormone to tell your gallbladder to contract. The lack of contraction ability can be due to scarring in the gallbladder from gallstones or inappropriate hormone signals.

Gallstones form when too much cholesterol and/or bilirubin (a breakdown product of red blood cells made by the liver) are present in the bile, or when the gallbladder does not contract and empty completely. Common risk factors include being overweight, eating a high-fat diet, eating a low-fat diet, and diabetes, but the hormone estrogen also makes gallstones more common in women than men. There are other risk factors as well. Gallstones may also be a cause of acute pancreatitis. Please see the section on that condition for more information.

One way to reduce the risk of gallstones may be through probiotics. Although probiotics have not been intensely studied for use in gallstone prevention, many strains are known to affect bile recirculation, cholesterol levels, and liver health, and thus can affect the amounts of bile and bilirubin that form the basis of gallstones. By doing so, probiotics can lessen the risk of gallstones.

26: REDUCES HEARTBURN TRIGGERS

You feel the burning sensation in your stomach and/or throat, burping, and sour taste. You knew you should not have eaten enchiladas, but the temptation was too great. You reach for an antacid medication and remind yourself to take your heartburn medication before eating enchiladas again.

Does this sound like something you do? Maybe your doctor prescribed heartburn medications, such as proton pump inhibitors or H2 blockers, to prevent heartburn, with no diagnosis as to why it happens. You may think the problem is overproduction of stomach acid, but that may not be the cause at all.

Heartburn, also called gastroesophageal reflux disease (GERD) or reflux, usually occurs when stomach contents sneak past the valve designed to keep them in the stomach and irritate the throat. Avoiding food and drink triggers and taking medications is the commonly prescribed advice. While those may stop the symptoms, the problem may or may not be the foods. The problem could stem from inflammation or dysfunction in your gastrointestinal (GI) tract.

When you eat, you should thoroughly chew food. Once swallowed, food goes down the esophagus and enters the stomach, small intestine, and then the colon before unused parts are expelled in feces. A problem anywhere in the GI tract can trigger heartburn.

Beneficial microbes such as probiotics line your entire GI tract and serve many functions, which include proper functioning of your GI tract, inflammation balance, improved digestion, and so on. Since different types of microbes typically live in the different places along the GI tract, with *Lactobacillus* usually along the length of the tract and *Bifidobacterium* primarily in the colon, different probiotics can help with heartburn depending where the problem originates. Rather than assuming acid overproduction is the problem, try balancing your gut microbiota with probiotics, and over time you may experience relief.

27: IMPROVES DIGESTION

All of us can use a little, or a lot of, help with digestion once in a while. If you experience chronic problems with digestion, however, you should see a gastroenterologist who can diagnose anything that might be seriously wrong.

Probiotics and raw fermented foods and drinks, such as sauerkraut and kefir that contain probiotic-like microbes, are very helpful for digestion. They help to keep your gastrointestinal tract at the proper pH for optimal digestion and help to break down foods. They also regulate the motion of your intestines so that food moves through at the proper pace.

The next time you need help with digestion, instead of reaching for a medication, try eating a spoonful (to start) of a raw fermented food or drink or taking a powdered probiotic supplement.

This is a basic sauerkraut recipe. You can experiment and add garlic, other vegetables, and spices like caraway or ginger to give it more depth of flavor.

4 cups shredded green cabbage
¾ teaspoon pink salt
Clean, wide-mouthed pint glass jar
1 large cabbage leaf
Washcloth or bandana
Rubber band

In a medium bowl, toss the shredded cabbage with the salt with clean hands, gently squeezing to draw out the juices.

Scoop handfuls of the mixture into the jar, packing it down as you go. Pour any juices from the bowl into the jar.

Fold the cabbage leaf and cover the top of the shredded cabbage mix, submerging the mix below the juice line.

Cover the top of the jar with a cloth and a rubber band.

Place jar in a warm place and begin tasting in about a week. Flavors develop over time, so cover with a lid and refrigerate when sauerkraut taste is to your liking. Add water to keep contents submerged.

28: HELPS IBS

It seems like one minute you have diarrhea (D) and the next minute you are constipated (C). Abdominal pain, cramping, and bloating come and go. You are tired of running to the bathroom frequently, or spending a long time in the bathroom waiting for something to happen. Irritable bowel syndrome (IBS) is a diagnosis of exclusion. Infections and other causes of your IBS-C dominant or IBS-D dominant symptoms have to be ruled out, but in many cases the diagnosis of IBS doesn't really provide answers. You may be on a low FODMAP (fermentable oligosaccharides, disaccharides, monosaccharides, and polyols) diet, which helps, but is restrictive.

Pinning down the exact causes of IBS is difficult because each person has his or her own combination of causes. One cause that is receiving much attention is that of a disrupted microbiome, as there is a strong association between having a gastrointestinal (GI) infection, like food poisoning, and the onset of IBS. Also, the FODMAP diet, and nonabsorbable antibiotics to kill gut microbiota, have provided relief in many patients, further supporting the suspicion of a disrupted microbiome as contributing to IBS.

Once the GI microbiome is disrupted, and especially if an infection is treated with antibiotics, it can take time for the resident microbiota to recover, if it ever does. A disrupted gut microbiome sets the stage for altered motility, intestinal hypersensitivity, gut immune activation, leaky gut, altered bile, mental disorders, and a host of other factors that can play a role in IBS. Probiotics, along with a proper diet, can help the GI tract get the microbes it needs to function normally.

PROBIOTIC YEAST MAY BE A HELP TOO

Both probiotic bacteria and yeasts have been effective in scientific trials for IBS. Work with a clinician to find the best probiotic supplement, along with diet and lifestyle factors, for you.

29: EASES INDIGESTION

Do you remember the Alka-Seltzer commercial with the man bemoaning, "I can't believe I ate the whole thing!"? That commercial captured the essence of indigestion, the uncomfortable feeling in the abdomen. Bloating, burping, heartburn, gas, and queasiness may be additional symptoms.

Indigestion literally means "not digestion." In other words, something along the way in your thirty-foot-long gastrointestinal (GI) tract is not working properly. It could be that you really did eat too much for your stomach to handle at once, so your stomach is stretched, causing discomfort. It could be that you didn't chew your food or you don't have enough stomach acid or digestive substances. Perhaps your gut motility is slow, you cannot absorb what you ate, or you are sensitive to the food you ate. These are just a few of the reasons why you could have indigestion. You can see that indigestion is not a diagnosis in itself.

Most people experience indigestion at one point or another, but if indigestion is a regular occurrence with you, instead of taking antacids and other medications to mask the symptoms, figure out *why* the indigestion is happening. Indigestion is a cry for help from your body.

One thing that can affect nearly every aforementioned cause is a disrupted gut microbiome. A variety of probiotics may be able to help correct the causes by rebalancing the gut microbiome, thereby improving stomach function, improving digestion and absorption, regulating gut motility, or preventing leaky gut and food sensitivity consequences.

PREVENTION IS KEY

Prevention is the key to alleviation of indigestion. Sometimes taking probiotics when faced with indigestion can help, but probiotics work best when used preventively. Add them to adequate amounts of nutritious food such as fermented vegetables to help propel food through your GI tract.

30: MAY REDUCE POSTSURGICAL INFECTIONS

You signed the waiver and were informed that postsurgical infections could occur after your surgery. While hospitals, outpatient centers, specialized treatment centers, and other sites where surgeries are performed do their best to reduce the chances of infection following surgery, the fact is that it is harder to do than it may seem.

Germs are nearly everywhere. Miss one tiny spot in cleaning, forget to let the cleaning solution sit long enough on a surface, or recirculate contaminated air in the surgical room, and germs multiply. Routinely killing all germs, or microorganisms, is usually not necessary, nor desirable. However, in the case of surgery, minimizing the risks of any kind of infection by reducing pathogenic or opportunistic microbes is of paramount importance.

Infections following surgeries do happen however, even with preventive antibiotics. The Centers for Disease Control and Prevention data show a surgical site infection (SSI) rate of just under 2 percent from 2006–2008. However, while that may seem low, the death rate of SSI is 3 percent, and 75 percent of those are directly attributable to the SSI. Prevention of SSIs is obviously not enough, but what can be done postsurgery?

After surgery, antibiotics are routinely prescribed to prevent bacterial infections. In the process, many beneficial bacteria may be killed, allowing the strongest bacteria, which are usually pathogenic, to survive and cause infections. The best thing to do postsurgery is to follow your doctor's instructions completely, supplementing with probiotics if permitted.

PREPARE YOUR SYSTEM BEFORE YOUR SURGERY

The best preventative measure to take prior to surgery is to prepare your body and immune system with oral probiotics and fermented foods, unless otherwise contraindicated, to make sure your gastrointestinal microbiome and your immune system are balanced and ready for the trauma of surgery and the chances of infection.

31: ENHANCES FEMALE FERTILITY

Infertility is a problem with the ability to conceive a child, and can be from the mother's or father's dysfunction, or both. At least one-third of infertility problems are from the female's perspective, with another one-third a combination from both sexes. An estimated 10–18 percent of couples experience infertility, and it can be devastating.

Major risk factors for female infertility are age, smoking, over- or underweight, alcohol indulgence, and a history of STDs (sexually transmitted diseases). As shown in other sections in this book, probiotics can help with weight issues, alcohol detoxification, and infections such as STDs. Out of the five major risk factors, you have control over four of them with your dietary and lifestyle choices. But what if none of those factors apply to you?

The process of creating a child, from conception to delivery, is complicated and can involve many factors, but when problems arise during or shortly after conception attempts, often the problem is hormonal. A woman has to be producing and releasing an egg from an ovary. If the egg is fertilized, it must travel down to the uterus and implant in the uterus. Both processes involve hormones. Maintaining the pregnancy also involves hormones.

Hormonal imbalances can be caused by polycystic ovary syndrome; premature ovarian function, which can be related to an autoimmune response; dysfunctions in the hypothalamus/pituitary glands, which are responsible for pregnancy-related hormones; and exposures to environmental toxins.

Probiotics can help with hormonal imbalances that might affect female fertility. By regulating bowel function; modulating immune function; reducing oxidative stress and inflammation to protect the brain, liver, and other organs; and breaking down toxins, many different species of probiotics may help balance your hormones so your dream of being a mother may come true.

32: ENHANCES MALE FERTILITY

Infertility is a problem with the ability to conceive a child, and can be from the mother's or father's dysfunction, or both. At least one-third of infertility problems are from the male's perspective, and some estimates are up to one-half.

Male infertility is due to low sperm production, sperm production abnormalities, or blockages that prevent sperm evacuation during ejaculation. Known causes weigh heavily on life choices such as diet and lifestyle, with other causes of illnesses, injuries, and chronic health conditions playing roles in some cases. Some of those causes may have no treatment, but dietary and lifestyle factors are under your control.

Male fertility is complex. You have to be able to produce healthy sperm that are able to move and function properly, have those sperm enter semen in high enough counts, and have erections to deliver the sperm. Hormone levels, cardiovascular disease, infections, diabetes, surgeries, autoimmune disease, medications and drugs, cancers, tumors, chemical and heavy metal exposure, weight, stress, and smoking and alcohol use are all factors that can affect the process. Probiotics, as part of healthy life choices, can help with many of those factors, as other sections in this book illustrate.

Reducing the factors involved in male infertility that you can control will not happen overnight, but it is comforting to know that many of them are under your control. Using probiotics to help with those factors is doable and may be the easiest to accomplish.

INCREASE YOUR FERTILITY

Specific research into male fertility with probiotics shows that probiotics have the capability of significantly increasing testosterone levels, reducing injury to the testicles, and improving sperm health. Different *Lactobacillus* and *Bifidobacterium* species were studied.

33: BANISHES INTESTINAL CRAMPS

It may surprise you that your intestinal cramps may not be actual cramps, as in a muscle cramp like a charley horse, but instead are the sensation of pain in your stomach or anywhere below. You may feel or hear gurgling, feel indigestion, feel extremely bloated, or have general distress.

Now you know the technicality of intestinal cramps, but how do you prevent them? Well, that depends on what is causing them. Some causes originate in the gastrointestinal (GI) tract itself: for example, built-up pressure from gas from too much swallowed air, food you cannot digest, or gut bacteria; food poisoning or another GI infection; and/or inflammatory bowel disease or cancers. Other causes could be outside the GI tract.

Prevention is the key to experiencing good intestinal health. All of the different genera of probiotics can help in various ways to alleviate the potential for intestinal cramps. By regulating intestinal motility, keeping pathogens under control, balancing electrolytes in the GI tract, improving digestion and nutrient absorption, reducing inflammation in the GI tract as well as systemically (body-wide), interacting with your immune and nervous systems, and reducing substances that can be irritating to your GI tract, probiotics can be one of the best and easiest ways to stand up straight, intestinal-cramp-free.

IF THE PROBLEM PERSISTS, SEE A DOCTOR

The pain you are experiencing can originate in the GI tract, but can also be referred from a site or organ outside of the intestinal tract, such as the kidneys, bile ducts, gallbladder, lungs, pancreas, or other organs in or near the abdominal cavity. If intestinal cramps plague you routinely, please have an examination by a qualified healthcare professional to rule out any serious causes.

34: REDUCES KIDNEY BURDEN

If you suffer from chronic kidney disease (CKD), you have company all over the globe. Worldwide 10 percent of the population has CKD, and for those aged sixty-five to seventy-four the statistics are even gloomier with 20 percent of men and 25 percent of women having it.

Kidneys filter toxins out of the blood and package wastes in urine, but those are not their only functions. They also activate some hormones, are involved in blood pressure regulation, and serve still other unique uses. Prevention of CKD and end-stage renal disease (ESRD) is a worthwhile effort for everyone in order to avoid facing the risks of dialysis, kidney replacement, associated cardiovascular disease and osteoporosis, and possible death.

Most prevention and treatment recommendations for CKD include eating a low-protein diet, along with a lifestyle that supports health. After all, some of the major risk factors for CKD such as obesity, diabetes, and high blood pressure are mostly lifestyle related. These recommendations are valid, but omit one important variable, gut health.

An imbalance in your gut microbiota can cause increased toxins in the bloodstream that your kidneys then have to filter, as well as inflammatory molecules that damage the kidneys. Probiotics can reduce the burden on your kidneys, thus allowing them to function better. For best results, balance your gut microbiota with the help of probiotics *before* you have kidney problems.

PROBIOTIC SUPPLEMENT TO NOTE

One probiotic product on the market for kidney health is Renadyl from Kibow Biotech. Kibow holds the registered trademark for the term "Enteric Dialysis" for Renadyl because it has shown efficacy in reducing the burden on the kidneys. It contains three researched strains: *Streptococcus thermophilus* KB-19, *Lactobacillus acidophilus* KB-27, and *Bifidobacterium longum* KB-31.

35: LESSENS RISK OF KIDNEY STONES

You may feel fine, and then all of a sudden a sharp pain hits in your lower back or abdomen. The pain may be intermittent, or it may radiate, or even stop. The cause? You may have kidney stones. You could even have kidney stones and not feel any pain.

According to a study in the United States in 2012, kidney stone prevalence was nearly 11 percent in men and 7 percent in women, with obese people suffering nearly twice as much as normal-weight individuals. Even children may suffer from kidney stones.

Kidney stone formation is complex and requires the necessary ingredients merging under the right conditions. Most kidney stones (80 percent) are made of calcium oxalate. Oxalates in the body are derived from three main sources: diet, normal human metabolism, and the breakdown of ascorbic acid. The main pathway to its elimination from the body is through urinary excretion, which involves the kidneys. Unfortunately, humans lack the enzymes needed to break down oxalates.

People at risk of kidney stone formation are often advised to avoid foods high in oxalates such as spinach, beet greens, nuts, beans, grains, cocoa, rhubarb, fruits, and others to decrease the load of oxalate absorption. However, avoidance of all oxalate-containing foods may not be practical due to the widespread prevalence of oxalates and the risk of malnutrition. The good news is that oxalate absorption from the gastrointestinal tract can be decreased with the help of probiotics.

PROBIOTICS CAN HELP

Probiotics can decrease oxalate absorption through proper elimination time and oxalate degradation. While the main oxalate-degrading bacterium is *Oxalobacter formigenes*, many species of probiotic bacteria, such as *Lactobacillus, Bifidobacterium,* and *Streptococcus thermophilus*, also have oxalate-degradation ability. Keeping your gut microbiota balanced through the intake and nurturing of probiotics can help reduce your chances of kidney stone formation.

36: IMPROVES LACTOSE INTOLERANCE

Not a serious health threat in itself, lactose intolerance produces symptoms of smelly gas, bloating, intestinal gurgling, and possible headache and diarrhea, depending on the amount of lactose ingested.

Lactose is a two-part sugar found in dairy products. It is usually broken down by a brush-border enzyme, lactase, in your small intestine, but some people do not have the capability to do that due to genetics, intestinal injuries, or disease. Also, humans typically lose the ability to break down lactose as they no longer rely on their mother's breast milk. The lactose then passes into the colon where resident microbes ferment it, resulting in the symptoms.

Lactose-free milk products are processed with lactase to degrade the natural lactose. Do you know the source of this lactase? In most cases, the commercial sources are yeasts because certain yeasts can produce large quantities of the enzyme.

Many of your gut microbes are capable of digesting lactose too. In fact, many of them prefer lactose as their first source of energy. Probiotic bacteria such as *Streptococcus thermophilus*, *Lactobacillus bulgaricus*, and several *Bifidobacterium* prefer lactose as well. Additionally, probiotics such as these can help prevent leaky gut and help repair it so that your body's ability to produce lactase may be restored.

MAINTAIN YOUR THRESHOLD

Lactose intolerance is not funny to those who suffer from it, but probiotics can help with it. You can take probiotics preventively to not only degrade lactose, but also to keep your gut intact. But keep in mind, you should not exceed the threshold at which your body can deal with lactose, even when using probiotics.

37: PROTECTS LIVER FUNCTION

Cooked liver may be one of the worst dinners you can remember from your childhood. Liver has a texture that is, well, interesting. If sourced from animals treated humanely, liver can be nutritious with high levels of vitamin A, iron and other minerals, B vitamins, and protein.

The reason liver is so nutritious is that it stores vitamins and minerals, and processes nutrients from foods you eat. It also performs other critical functions such as controlling amounts of nutrients in the blood, providing enzymes for detoxification, assembling proteins, producing cholesterol and bile, and converting some hormones into active forms.

Your liver is a large organ in the upper right front quadrant of your abdomen, tucked mostly behind your ribs. It is your main detoxification organ inside your body, and as such it deals with a lot of toxins and free-radical buildup during its normal activities. These free radicals, part of oxidative stress, can damage your liver if they exceed your body's capacity to neutralize them with antioxidants.

Injury to and infection in your liver affects your overall health and subjects your liver to increased oxidative stress.

One way to decrease the stress load is to minimize the toxins and inflammatory molecules that pass from your intestines through the portal vein to the liver. Probiotics of many types can help with this. By reducing pathogens that produce toxins and inflammatory molecules, probiotics spare the liver from unnecessary assaults. Additionally, by helping the bowels function normally, bodily wastes and excess hormones are eliminated instead of being reabsorbed and sent to the liver.

DON'T WAIT UNTIL TROUBLE ARISES

Don't wait for your liver function to be compromised. Protect your liver by keeping your gut microbiota balanced with probiotics!

38: MAY REDUCE RISK OF NAFLD

Your liver is an important organ in your body, and it functions best without excess levels of fat in it. It is normal to have some fat in your liver, since your liver assembles cholesterol and fatty acids for your body's needs. In NAFLD, nonalcoholic fatty liver disease, fat levels build up to the point that they impair the functioning of the liver. It doesn't take a lot of extra fat to impair your liver; 5–10 percent of extra fat will do it.

In the past, people thought that only alcoholics suffered from hepatic steatosis, fat buildup in the liver, but more than 30 percent of US adults have NAFLD. In addition to decreasing your liver's ability to function, NAFLD can lead to scarring of the liver (cirrhosis), liver failure, and liver cancer.

Risk factors for NAFLD are being overweight or obese, having type 2 diabetes, and dysregulation of blood lipids, especially with high triglycerides and low HDL. Diet and lifestyle obviously play important roles in the development and persistence of NAFLD. Additionally, gut health plays a significant role.

Your gut microbiota can either be in a balanced state or a state of dysbiosis, or microbial imbalance. Dysbiosis results in toxins and chemicals that ultimately have to be eliminated through feces or detoxed by your liver. This puts added stress on your liver and hinders its ability to do its job, allowing fats to accumulate. Probiotics help correct dysbiosis and lessen your risk of NAFLD.

TO MAKE A BEET KVASS FOR LIVER HEALTH, FOLLOW THESE INSTRUCTIONS

Beets are cleansing to the liver. Fermenting them adds the benefits of beneficial microbes. Drink the juice and eat the beets in this recipe.

3 medium organic beets
Clean, wide-mouthed pint glass jar
2 teaspoons pink salt
Filtered water
Washcloth or bandana and rubber band

Scrub, then dice beets and place them in the jar.

Mix salt in water and pour over beets.

Cover jar with washcloth and rubber band and begin checking in three days. You may add other vegetables or herbs scuh as caraway or ginger for added flavor.

39: MAY HELP PREVENT CONDITIONS LEADING TO LYMPHOMA

Lymphoma is not one single type of cancer, but all types of it develop in the immune/lymphatic system. One of the scariest things about lymphoma is that it happens in the very body system that is designed to protect you against cancers.

The function of your lymphatics are to drain fluids and wastes from cells, transport lipids (types of fat) from your gastrointestinal (GI) tract to the blood, and carry out immune responses. Your lymph nodes are masses of tissue that store immune cells, and filter and destroy pathogens and abnormal cells from your lymph fluid to decrease threats to you. When you are fighting an infection, your lymph nodes in certain areas may enlarge and be tender. Once the infection is under control, lymph nodes should return to their normal size. If they do not, that could be one indication of a tumor as lymphoma.

Although research into the link between lymphoma and the gut microbiome is in its infancy, one link that has shown validity in mice is that the gut microbiome can induce genetic mutations in the GI tract via oxidative stress and inflammatory assaults. These mutations are caused by pathogens, creating a toxic environment in the intestines that can spread throughout the body.

All types of probiotics work to reduce the pathogens that produce toxic substances that cause oxidative stress and inflammation. Many probiotics can help regulate the inflammatory response, inducing anti-inflammatory responses in cells that would otherwise be in chronic inflammation mode.

While they are not a proven preventative of or a cure in themselves of lymphoma, probiotics may work to counteract some of the variables that can contribute to lymphoma.

CAUTION: DO NOT SELF-TREAT!

If you have or suspect you have lymphoma, please seek appropriate medical care. Probiotics should not be used as a standalone treatment against lymphoma.

40: PROMOTES EYE HEALTH

Macular degeneration (MD) is a major cause of central-vision loss in people age fifty-five and older. Causes include age-related changes, genetic variations, and lifestyle factors contributing to inflammation such as smoking, alcohol use, sunlight exposure, nutrient-poor diet, and medications.

The macula is a specialized part of the retina in the back of the eye responsible for central vision, sharpness in images seen, and recognition of color differences. Carotenoids, such as lutein, zeaxanthin, and meso-zeaxanthin, are concentrated there and play important roles in the structure and function of the macula, including providing protection of the retina from light-induced oxidative stress damage from free radicals.

Some studies show that a diet high in carotenoids can partially reverse some of the functions lost due to MD, so increasing foods like dark green leafy vegetables can turn a nutrient-poor diet, which can be a cause of MD, to a nutrient-rich diet, which prevents or improves MD. In order to absorb lutein and zeaxanthin, the cells lining the intestines must be healthy.

Probiotics of many types work to keep intestinal cells healthy by protecting them from invasive pathogens and their toxic products, by keeping the cells close together so they maintain integrity, by producing short-chain fatty acids that nourish the cells, by producing anti-inflammatory chemicals to reduce inflammation in intestinal tissue, and by communicating with your genes to effect an appropriate immune response to contents in the gastrointestinal tract.

PROBIOTICS PROMOTE EYE HEALTH

At this time, there is not a specific probiotic that is recommended to directly influence the development and progression of macular degeneration. However, the fact that probiotics promote eye health by quelling inflammation, and influencing the digestion and absorption of carotenoids, suggests that probiotics can play a supplementary role in MD prevention and therapy.

41: DECREASES VAGINAL DRYNESS

Jokes are commonly made about women in the transition to menopause, but there is nothing funny about night sweats that disturb sleep, mood swings, vaginal dryness, and decreased sex drive. Menopause signals the end of a woman's fertility and reproductive capability, and while it can mean freedom from menstruation and pregnancy, it can also bring a sense of loss, especially if it was abruptly induced as a result of surgery.

When a woman's ovaries stop producing estrogen and progesterone, her body has to learn how to manage without higher amounts of those hormones. Other tissues make those hormones, but not to the extent of the ovaries. Among the menopausal symptoms, one that clearly is associated with a disruption in vaginal microbiota is vaginal dryness.

Vaginal dryness is associated with vulvovaginal atrophy (shrinkage), reduced vaginal secretions, and decreased production of glycogen by vaginal cells that serves as an energy source for microbes. Studies show that when estrogen declines, the vaginal microbiome changes, with a decrease in relative amounts of the *Lactobacillus* species. Supplementation with estrogen is typified by an increase in the relative amounts of *Lactobacillus*, along with an improvement in vaginal dryness and its associations.

Many researchers believe that probiotics such as the *Lactobacillus* species not only are influenced by changes in the vagina caused by changes in hormone levels, but that they can also influence which changes occur. Routine supplementation with probiotics may be able to prevent vulvovaginal atrophy from occurring, at least as drastically as it occurs in menopause.

42: OFFERS HELP FOR MS SYMPTOMS

Multiple sclerosis (MS) involves the central nervous system and how information is processed in the brain and communicated to the body. Most people are twenty to fifty years old when diagnosed, more women than men are affected, and no two people have the exact same journey with the disease. While the exact causes are not known, autoimmunity, a situation in which the body attacks cells that it mistakenly believes are foreign, is believed to be one of the main causes.

More common symptoms of MS are fatigue, numbness or tingling, weakness, vision problems, dizziness or a sensation of spinning of surroundings, walking difficulties, spastic muscle movements, pain, bladder problems, bowel problems, sexual problems, cognitive problems, depression, and emotional instability. There are a host of less common symptoms, and symptoms that are comorbid with other conditions, making it difficult to distinguish in the beginning.

MS is a very complicated disease, and it is no wonder that treatment regimens differ depending on the individual's circumstances and the progression of the disease. However, probiotics offer help for MS symptoms.

Probiotics are known to interact with the body's immune system and may help with an imbalance like autoimmunity. Additionally, probiotics can regulate bowel function, assist in clearing infections of some pathogens in the gastrointestinal tract, and provide digestion and nutrient absorption assistance. Probiotics also help with brain fog, poor concentration, depression, anxiety, and irritability that are common in MS. Talk to your healthcare provider to see if probiotics can help you in your treatment plan.

43: LESSENS NEC RISK

Necrotizing enterocolitis (NEC) is a serious gastrointestinal (GI) disorder that frequently affects premature newborns. It results in a diseased state in which intestinal tissue becomes damaged and dies, has a high surgery rate (nearly 50 percent), and has a high rate of mortality, especially in very low birth weight infants. NEC affects approximately 7 percent of all very low birth weight infants and carries a death rate greater than 20 percent.

The exact causes of NEC are unknown, but it is suspected that it is related to multiple factors such as genetic susceptibility, prematurity, formula feeding, and gut dysbiosis (disruption in normal flora). In fact, studies show that preterm infants have lower levels of protective *Lactobacillus* and *Bifidobacterium* species compared to full-term infants. Probiotics of many types can help with gut dysbiosis by keeping pathogens under control by producing acids and antimicrobials, by crowding them out, by preventing attachment to gut tissue, and by displacing them if they do become attached. In doing so, toxic products from the pathogens are reduced. Probiotics also help maintain intestinal-barrier function, assist in proper development and functioning of the intestines, and help with nutrient digestion and absorption.

It is also known that the immune system in premature babies is immature. Probiotics communicate with the body's immune system for proper development and regulation of the immune system.

Although there are no official recommendations yet as to probiotic strains or dosages to be given to infants at risk of NEC, trials with probiotics show that NEC is significantly reduced in infants who received a multispecies probiotic supplement compared to those who did not.

44: HELPS REDUCE RISK OF ACUTE PANCREATITIS

Pancreatitis is inflammation of the pancreas. It can develop slowly over time or happen acutely, meaning intensely and abruptly. Symptoms of acute pancreatitis (AP) range from being mild to life-threatening, and include pain and swelling in the upper left side of the abdomen that may radiate into the back, nausea, vomiting, burping, fever, and increased heart rate.

Most cases of AP are caused by gallstones (please see section on gallstones) or heavy alcohol consumption. Trauma, infections, medications, surgery, and inherited metabolic disorders are other causes, but in some cases the exact cause is unknown.

Most people associate the pancreas with insulin secretion, but it also secretes other hormones and pancreatic juice containing digestive enzymes, so dysfunction in the pancreas affects the entire body. In the gut, without adequate pancreatic juice, the small intestine becomes susceptible to tissue injury and overgrowth from pathogens. This situation creates a risk of infection from bacteria that translocate from the gut to the pancreas, as well as a risk of more oxidative stress to the pancreas caused by toxins released from the pathogens.

Probiotics such as *Lactobacillus*, *Lactococcus*, and *Bifidobacterium* species used in animal studies show that probiotics act preventively to reduce the severity of pancreatic injury and act therapeutically to reduce pancreatic cell oxidative stress and cell death in AP.

PREVENTION IS KEY

The important point to be noted is that, as seen in many other conditions highlighted in this book, the value of probiotics really stands out in prevention. While probiotics can be useful as therapy for established conditions, keeping your body healthier with the use of probiotics prophylactically carries few risks for most people with many benefits.

45: BATTLES PERIODONTAL DISEASE

Your teeth were cleaned, your gums prodded, and now you feel like someone hit you in the mouth. Is an overenthusiastic dental hygienist to blame? Perhaps, but you may have been told that you have periodontal disease (PD). PD can range from gum inflammation to serious infection affecting gum tissue and the bones that support the teeth.

How did this happen? Bacteria and yeasts in your mouth coexist with saliva and other substances in your mouth, but they do not live in isolation. Instead, they form protective biofilms, colonies of different microbes in which their survival is enhanced by sharing of resources. One such biofilm in your mouth is plaque, which is why you have to brush your teeth in order to break it up. If plaque stays undisturbed, it forms tartar, which then requires professional cleaning to remove.

In PD, gums pull away from the teeth forming pockets that provide the perfect breeding ground for microbes such as *Porphyromonas gingivalis* that cause infection. If PD progresses, tooth loss may occur. Aside from the aesthetics of PD, a major concern is what those oral pathogens are doing to the rest of your body, as PD is associated with a greater risk of cardiovascular disease, and particularly heart attacks, as well as other health problems.

Along with better oral hygiene and a more nutritious diet to provide nutrients that support gum and tooth health, probiotics can help in the prevention and serve as additional therapy in PD.

PROBIOTICS IN ORAL HEALTH PRODUCTS

There are many oral health probiotic products on the market today, from lozenges to oral supplements to toothpastes and mouth rinses. One of the probiotic genera that is commonly found in these products is *Lactobacillus*, because *Lactobacillus* bacteria have the capability to integrate into biofilms such as plaque and disrupt them.

46: EASES PMS

Emotional and behavioral symptoms such as angry outbursts, depression, irritability, crying spells, anxiety, poor concentration, social withdrawal, sleep disturbances, and changes in eating and drinking patterns, as well as physical symptoms such as breast tenderness, bloating, headache, water retention, and pains, are common with premenstrual syndrome (PMS). Estimates are that 75–90 percent of menstruating women experience at least one symptom of PMS during the two weeks prior to menstruation.

The exact cause of PMS is unknown, but nutritional deficiencies, inflammation and oxidative stress, and hormonal imbalances are suspected causes. There most likely are several factors involved, and those factors may vary from month to month, making PMS resolution a difficult target to hit. Antidepressants may help some of the emotional and behavioral symptoms, and analgesics such as acetaminophen may relieve some of the physical symptoms, but neither is addressing the causes.

Your gut microbiome and probiotics can impact all of the suspected causes. As long as you eat nutritious food, probiotics can assist in digestion, making food nutrients, including vitamins,

minerals, and antioxidants (which are critical to quell oxidative stress), more available to you. Probiotics can also help with absorption of those nutrients.

Probiotics have the capability to reduce inflammation and oxidative stress, both locally and systemically (body-wide) by influencing your immune system and the genes involved in inflammation. Probiotics can also influence hormonal imbalances via various mechanisms to address your PMS symptoms.

HELP TO FEEL NORMAL AGAIN

There is no magic pill to rid you of all of your PMS symptoms, but balancing your gut microbiome with probiotics and probiotic-enhancing foods is a great way to address some of the causes, instead of only the symptoms, to help you feel like your normal self again.

47: IMPEDES PNEUMONIA PATHOGENS

Pneumonia is an infection that causes inflammation, often with fluid or pus buildup, in the air sacs of one or both lungs and can be bacterial, viral, or fungal in origin. Pneumonia may be a mild infection in some people, but it is one of the top infections that leads to death in immunocompromised people. Children younger than two years old, adults older than sixty-five, and persons with a weakened immune system from disease (like HIV), chemotherapy, or medications that suppress the immune system are at highest risk.

Knowledge of the organism(s) involved is critical so that appropriate treatment can be prescribed, but it can be difficult to discern exactly which microbe is at fault, especially in bacterial pneumonia. Pathogenic bacteria such as *Streptococcus pneumoniae*, or bacteria in the *Klebsiella*, *Pseudomonas*, or *Mycoplasma* genera, are typical causes of bacterial pneumonia.

As with many conditions, research into the lung microbiome during health and infection, and trials with probiotics for prevention or treatment of the various forms of pneumonia, are in their infancy. Numerous probiotics are being investigated in animal models and human trials to determine which ones are the most effective for various scenarios. You may be surprised to know that although pneumonia occurs in the lungs, it increases intestinal permeability (leaky gut), and much of the benefit of oral probiotics seen thus far is from the maintenance of the intestinal barrier so that the production and circulation of pro-inflammatory chemicals is reduced and immune function is restored.

Although probiotics have many ways of inhibiting the growth of or killing pathogens, they do not act like most drugs, with only one mode of operation. They also work best preventively, so keeping your intestinal tract healthy and balanced with probiotics can help prevent leaky gut and an uncontrolled, damaging inflammatory response to pathogens.

48: FIGHTS POUCHITIS

Pouchitis is inflammation of the pouch, formed from surgery to remove the colon and rectum, which connects the last section of the small intestine to the anus. This pouch serves as a reservoir to store and eliminate stools in the place of the colon and rectum. Pouchitis can cause more frequent and possibly more strained bowel movements, abdominal bloating, cramping or pain, and sometimes blood in the stool. Fever and other signs of severe infection are possible.

All cases of pouchitis should be diagnosed and treated by a qualified physician. Up to 40 percent of patients who have had this surgery develop pouchitis every year, with the typical treatment consisting of a fourteen-day course of antibiotics. It is not uncommon for infection to relapse. Sometimes that occurs because of antibiotic-resistant bacteria, but polyps, NSAID (nonsteroidal anti-inflammatory drug) use, autoimmune disease, and reduced blood flow to the pouch are among other causes of relapse.

Institutions such as the Cleveland Clinic recognize the importance of probiotics when antibiotics are prescribed and state that the doctor may also recommend strains of *Lactobacillus, Bifidobacterium,* or *Streptococcus thermophilus* for pouchitis. One medical food-grade probiotic supplement, VSL#3, has the distinction of being able to advertise its use as a treatment for pouchitis. This supplement contains eight different strains of *Bifidobacterium, Lactobacillus,* and *Streptococcus thermophilus.* The most potent form is available by prescription only (in the United States).

TALK TO YOUR DOCTOR ABOUT ADDING PROBIOTICS

Remember, pouchitis is a condition that should be evaluated and treated by a qualified physician. He/she may recommend probiotics, depending on your health status, as a means to reduce relapse rates and prevent complications from antibiotics.

49: REDUCES RISK OF PRETERM BIRTH

The upcoming birth of a baby is an exciting time, but when the baby is born prematurely, at less than thirty-seven weeks of gestation, concerns arise for the health of the newborn. The extra three weeks in the womb are important for full development of most body systems, particularly the respiratory (lungs), cardiovascular (heart and blood pressure), nervous (brain), gastrointestinal (digestion, absorption, and liver), and immune systems.

There are many risk factors for PB, such as multiple fetuses, high blood pressure, poor nutrition, smoking, stress, and so on, but the ones that microbiome researchers are most interested in are infections and local/systemic (body-wide) inflammation. Infections cause an immune response with associated inflammation, which can destabilize pregnancy. Infectious microbes and/or inflammatory molecules can travel systemically from one place in the body causing problems in other sites.

Research shows that there is a relationship between PB and inflammation/infections, such as kidney infections, pneumonia, periodontal disease, bacterial infections in the uterus, and pathogens in amniotic fluid, the amniotic sac, or the placenta. Exactly how the pathogens end up in the fetal environment is not currently known, but one theory is that pathogens involved in bacterial vaginosis (see bacterial vaginosis section) ascend into the vagina, go through the cervix, and enter the uterus.

As other sections in this book show, an imbalance in the gut and/or lung, oral, and vaginal microbiomes is associated with those conditions. Probiotics can help resolve those conditions, and in doing so, can reduce the risk for PB.

PREVENTION

Probiotics help prevent infections and inflammation, which can cause PB. While it is best to balance your gut and vaginal microbiomes and heal a leaky gut prior to becoming pregnant, probiotics may be helpful during pregnancy. Discuss your situation with your healthcare provider to see if probiotics may reduce your risks of preterm delivery.

50: ADDRESSES RADIATION ENTERITIS

Radiation is used as a treatment modality in many cancers. The gastrointestinal (GI) tract is very sensitive to the effects of radiation, resulting in irritation and inflammation of the small and large intestines in the condition called radiation enteritis (RE). RE can occur right after the first radiation treatment or within eight weeks thereafter, as acute RE, but some people will suffer with longer-term RE.

Symptoms of RE can include nausea, vomiting, abdominal cramping, diarrhea, persistent urges to have bowel movements, discharge of mucus, pain, itching, and/or bleeding. Current treatments consist of rehydration, low-fat and low-fiber diet, antidiarrheal drugs, pain relievers, steroids to reduce inflammation, and possible surgery. Unfortunately, none of those treatments addresses the underlying causes of the inflammation, nor do they assist the GI tract in its repair so that it can return to normal functioning, without invasive measures.

There are not many clinical trials using probiotics in the prevention or treatment of RE, but the results are encouraging. Probiotics work by affecting the immune system and inflammation, protecting intestinal cells from pathogenic assaults, nourishing intestinal cells, aiding digestion and nutrient absorption, balancing electrolytes, regulating bowel movements, and keeping mucus and intestinal cells intact. In doing those things, they hold much promise for prevention and treatment of RE.

TALK WITH YOUR DOCTOR

If you know you are undergoing radiation or already have undergone it, talk to your qualified healthcare professional about the use of probiotics and other gut-healing measures with your current state of health.

The word *rotavirus* can bring up images of horror if you have ever watched one of your children rapidly dehydrate from it. Rotavirus is an infection that can go from being a nuisance to life-threatening in a matter of hours, especially in young children who can become severely dehydrated very quickly.

Rotavirus is a viral disease that causes stomach and intestinal inflammation, with symptoms of explosive, watery diarrhea, likely with vomiting, fever, and abdominal pain. The virus is shed in stool, so proper hand washing and washing of toys, bed linens, and so on are important to minimize risk of transmission, but someone could be infected for up to two days before he or she presents with symptoms, unknowingly transmitting the virus to others. Conventional treatments consist of keeping the patient hydrated via oral or intravenous electrolyte solutions until the symptoms pass in a few days.

Although there are vaccinations for rotavirus, it is possible for a vaccinated person, or a person who once had rotavirus, to become sick from the virus again because there are different strains of the virus. Since there are different strains, the best thing to do is to have an immune system capable of quickly fighting the virus.

Probiotics have a place in immune function and in prevention of and/or therapy for rotavirus. Since 70 percent or more of the immune system is in the gastrointestinal tract, oral probiotics have both direct and indirect communication with the immune system. Most studies on rotavirus were performed in animals, but results show that several *Lactobacillus* and *Bifidobacterium* strains are capable of reducing the duration of diarrhea, reducing intestinal inflammation, and increasing rotavirus-specific antibodies during infection. Probiotics also lessen the rotavirus's impact and can be taken before, during, and after experiencing symptoms.

PREVENTION VERSUS THERAPY

Prevention is always preferable to therapy during an active infection. Probiotics can be helpful for both in rotavirus. Probiotics work best preventively to help with microbial variety in the gut.

52: IMPROVES SHORT-BOWEL SYNDROME

Sometimes people have to have massive bowel reconstruction surgery with removal of a significant portion of their small intestine, and possibly part or all of their large intestine. This could be due to intestinal diseases like Crohn's disease, trauma to the bowel, surgery, cancer treatment, or a genetic or developmental malfunction in the small intestine. What results is poor absorption of nutrients like vitamins, minerals, protein, fat, water, and others in a condition called short-bowel syndrome (SBS).

SBS is relatively rare, but the main symptom is watery diarrhea. Bloating, cramping, fatigue, foul gas and stools, heartburn, vomiting, and weakness are other symptoms. SBS can result in malnutrition and complications of ulcers, kidney stones, and SIBO (small intestinal bacterial overgrowth). The main treatments are nutritional and hydration support, but the complications require other therapies. Antibiotics are frequently prescribed to treat SIBO.

The human body is amazing, however, and sometimes the small intestine in young children can grow to replace some of the missing intestine. Sometimes simply introducing the correct probiotic supplement can improve SBS and ease some of its complications. In one case study in a young child with SBS and SIBO, *Bifidobacterium breve* Yakult, *Lactobacillus casei* Shirota, and a prebiotic substance dramatically improved her nutritional status, intestinal function, and intestinal movement (motility).

Probiotics such as those can improve SBS by protecting and nourishing intestinal cells, combatting pathogens, restoring intestinal motility, improving digestion and absorption, affecting bile, and balancing the immune system, among others.

DO NOT SELF-TREAT SBS

Since SBS can lead to sepsis, a violent immune response to bacteria in the bloodstream, SBS must be evaluated by a qualified physician. If you are at risk of SBS, please speak to your qualified physician about the potential to use probiotics as a preventative measure or as part of a treatment plan.

53: PROMOTES SINUS HEALTH

Do you have a chronically stuffed up nose? Have you had multiple sinus infections or sinus surgeries? If so, then you have had some sort of chronic rhinosinusitis (CRS) and you know how painful your sinuses and your head can feel.

Your sinuses are air-filled cavities around your nose and eyes. Their main theorized purpose is to help filter, humidify, and warm air you breathe in before it gets to your lungs. The cavities are lined with soft tissue and mucus, and unsurprisingly, microbes.

Your sinuses are home to a diverse community of microbes ideally suited for living there. Under normal circumstances, they help to maintain the health of your sinuses. In CRS, the community is disrupted and proportions of inflammation-causing microbes tend to dominate. Studies so far show that there is not one single community present in the sinuses of healthy individuals or in individuals with CRS, but they do point to pathogens such as *Staphylococcus aureus* as being able to disrupt the microbial balance.

What disrupts balanced life in the sinuses? Sinus surgeries can, and products used intranasally (inside the nose) may, but evidence is pointing to antibiotic use as being the most influential factor. Antibiotics kill off many bacteria, but the survivors in both the gut and the nasal passages are usually tenacious pathogens, which then can dominate, causing inflammation.

As with other studies on body-area-specific microbiomes, research into the sinus microbiome is in its infancy, so no specific probiotics are recommended for CRS. However, since probiotics in general, when taken orally, can affect areas of the body far distances from the gut, restoring balance in the gut microbiome, especially after antibiotic use, may reduce inflammation in the sinuses and help your body to clear CRS and promote sinus health.

54: ENHANCES SPORTS PERFORMANCE

You push yourself: just one more mile, one more minute, or one more set. You know that in the end what you are doing is good, and necessary, for your health. And it is. Regular exercise benefits your physical, mental, and emotional health. However, it doesn't matter if you are a serious athlete or a weekend warrior, or someone in between; a good workout can leave you temporarily more susceptible to problems originating in your gastrointestinal (GI) tract.

Regular intense training, such as that undertaken by athletes, is often accompanied by fatigue, mood problems, GI distress, and an inability to perform at maximum capacity over time. These are all indications of an overload of stress. They are also why intense training must be fueled by nutritious food and followed by sufficient rest so that the brain and body can recuperate and avoid overtraining syndrome.

While stress can improve focus, strength, endurance, and agility, too much ends up breaking down the very things you are trying to build up. Intense training temporarily increases intestinal permeability, or leaky gut, so that toxins, other particles, and microbes are able to leave the intestines and enter body-wide circulation and cause inflammation in many body parts. Leaky gut also hinders your ability to absorb the very nutrients you need to fuel your workouts.

Probiotics of many kinds can help prevent leaky gut caused by stress, and can balance gut microbiota so that less inflammatory molecules are released into your circulation. The result is enhanced sports performance. Regardless of your level of activity, minding the health of your GI tract with nutritiously dense foods and beneficial microbes can help you avoid a prolonged postworkout leaky gut and its detrimental consequences.

55: LIMITS STOMACH FLU

You were fine one minute and the next minute you are running to the bathroom with diarrhea, bending over with abdominal pain, feeling nauseated, and possibly even vomiting or experiencing a fever and achiness. Was it something you ate or drank, or did? While it could be related to food poisoning, it also could be caused by a virus.

Viral gastroenteritis (VG), often called the stomach flu, does not really happen in your stomach and it is not caused by a flu virus. Flu viruses are respiratory viruses, whereas intestinal viruses are enteroviruses. VG is caused by a type of enterovirus that infects your small intestine. It is usually spread by food, drink, utensils, stool, and saliva contaminated with the virus. Raw shellfish may also harbor enteroviruses. Since VG normally takes a day or two to incubate before symptoms are felt, it can be difficult, if not impossible, to trace the origin.

Notorious viruses known to cause VG are norovirus and rotavirus. The main risk with VG is that of dehydration, so it is very important to stay hydrated and balance electrolytes with drinks such as broths, nonsugary electrolyte replacement drinks, and fresh vegetable juices. Normally the viral symptoms will end in a day or two.

Probiotics of many types may help in the prevention of the stomach flu by keeping the immune system balanced so that it recognizes an invader sooner and deals with it more effectively. Probiotics taken daily can protect the intestinal cells so that they maintain their integrity or quickly recover their integrity during VG. They can also help with electrolyte balance and motility in the intestines for diarrhea and dehydration management.

56: THWARTS STOMACH ULCERS

Many of the symptoms of a stomach ulcer (including feeling of fullness, bloating, burping, heartburn, and/or nausea) overlap with other gastrointestinal (GI) conditions, but the main discerning symptom is burning stomach pain. If you frequently reach for antacids, or need food in your stomach to feel less pain, you may have an ulcer. A gastroenterologist can diagnose ulcers.

Sometimes ulcers can occur on the inside of the upper portion of your small intestine, too, and together these duodenal ulcers and stomach (gastric) ulcers are called *peptic ulcers.* The most common causes of peptic ulcers are infection with the bacterium *H. pylori* and overuse of aspirin and other pain medications such as NSAIDs (nonsteroidal anti-inflammatory drugs), which block the stomach from being able to repair itself. Spicy foods and stress used to be blamed for peptic ulcers, but while those can certainly either contribute to the conditions that predispose you to ulcer development or make your symptoms worse, they in themselves are not to blame.

H. pylori is an interesting bacterium in that there is debate if it is a normal inhabitant of your stomach and only sometimes causes problems, or if it is a microbe that should be eliminated. Conventional treatment consists of antibiotics to kill the *H. pylori* and acid-blocking or neutralizing medication to reduce stomach acid so the lining can heal. However, many cases of *H. pylori* are resistant to antibiotics.

Numerous *Lactobacillus, Bacillus, Bifidobacterium,* and *Saccharomyces* probiotics have antagonistic abilities against *H. pylori* and are being tested in combination with conventional therapy. These probiotics, when given in addition to triple-antibiotic therapy, increase *H. pylori* elimination rates and decrease side effects from the antibiotic treatment. Probiotics can help you thwart attacks from the causes of stomach ulcers.

57: HELPS RESOLVE THYROID PROBLEMS

The thyroid is a gland in your neck. Its main function is to make hormones that are key regulators of your metabolism. Problems with it can affect every body part, with the most obvious symptom being changes in energy levels. The most common thyroid problem is an underactive thyroid in hypothyroidism caused by autoimmune Hashimoto's disease, thyroid removal, potentially lithium and iodide treatments, and an underconversion of inactive thyroid hormones (T4) to active ones (T3). There are other thyroid problems, too, such as an overactive thyroid caused by hyperthyroid autoimmune Grave's disease, thyroid nodules, cancers, pituitary gland malfunction, or inflammation of the thyroid.

The reasons behind thyroid malfunction are intricate and many, but autoimmunity and underconversion seem to dominate. Probiotics can affect immune function, so they can play a role in balancing out autoimmune imbalances, especially preventively. They also control pathogenic microbes that cause inflammatory molecules to leave the gut and affect other body parts, such as the thyroid and remote tissues, thus contributing to underconversion in remote tissues.

Thyroid hormones produced by the thyroid are carried bound to protiens in the bloodstream to body tissues. Some tissues convert T4 to T3, some are converted in the liver, and some are converted in the gastrointestinal (GI) tract by microbiota. If the gut is overpopulated by GI pathogens, the liver is not functioning well due to insults from GI pathogens, and other tissues are affected by the same insults, underconversion of T4 to T3 can occur, resulting in symptoms of hypothyroidism. In this case, thyroid function is not the problem and more detailed blood panel results are needed to determine the cause.

Probiotics can help resolve problems contributing to underconversion of hormones, autoimmunity, and inflammatory states so that thyroid hormones can work normally. See a qualified professional for help.

58: LESSENS TOXIC SHOCK SYNDROME RISK

Toxic shock syndrome (TSS) is a serious illness caused by infection in the bloodstream from the pathogen *Staphylococcus aureus* (*S. aureus*) and its production of toxic shock syndrome toxin-1. The infection causes systemic (body-wide) immune activation and inflammation and can lead to organ failure and death.

TSS affects high numbers of premenopausal women in developed countries and is usually associated with tampon use, but it can also be linked to surgery and open wounds. *S. aureus* is usually found on the outside of the body, but insertion of tampons increases the risk of its translocation into the vagina. When tampons are left in place too long, the conditions favorable to the growth of *S. aureus* develop, allowing this pathogen to overtake the normal defenses of the vagina and enter the bloodstream.

Lactobacillus species of bacteria are usually the dominant bacteria in the vagina, making conditions inhospitable to pathogens such as *S. aureus*. During menstruation, however, the pH of the vagina changes from a low pH to a higher pH due to blood flow, favoring the growth of pathogens.

Prevention of TSS from tampon use involves removing the tampon at or before the manufacturer-recommended intervals for the tampon, and keeping your vaginal microbiota balanced. Probiotics, heavily weighted with the *Lactobacillus* species, taken internally or inserted vaginally, can help balance the vaginal microbiome.

Some of the symptoms of TSS are sudden fever and flu-like aches, which can be caused by many illnesses. However, if you have been using tampons, and especially super absorbent tampons, and develop a sudden fever, it is critical that you seek emergency help.

SEEK HELP IMMEDIATELY

Toxic shock syndrome is a very serious illness that can lead to death if not promptly addressed. It is critical that you seek immediate medical help if you suspect TSS.

59: HELPS CONSEQUENCES OF MAJOR PHYSICAL TRAUMA

Major trauma (MT) is injury caused by physical harm to an individual that has the possibility of death or disability. Burns, motor vehicle accidents, assaults, surgeries, and falls are common causes of MT. Many people may not view concussions as MT, but traumatic brain injuries like concussions can indeed be MT.

One of the things that all types of MT have in common is that they result in extreme stress to the body, and in turn to intestinal permeability. Intestinal cells should be close together and selective about the kinds of substances that are permitted to pass inside or between them. In intestinal permeability, or leaky gut, the intestinal cells develop gaps in between them, allowing bacteria and toxins, which should remain in the intestines, to enter the bloodstream and cause injury to the brain, organs, and body systems. Sepsis, or infection in the blood, is a life-threatening condition caused by bacterial translocation, but there can be milder forms of bacterial translocation problems such as mood changes, cognition problems, liver dysfunction, and so on.

Stress in itself causes an imbalance in the microbiota in the gut, with many pathogens favored in an environment washed in stress hormones. The pathogens are able to overpower the beneficial microbes that normally keep pathogens under control and disrupt the structure and functions of the intestines.

If not contraindicated, probiotics may play a role in MT by boosting the effects of beneficial microbes in the gut to maintain a secure intestinal barrier and control pathogens. They also can help the body extract more nutrients from foods and drinks to help the body heal.

DO NOT SELF-TREAT MT

Any MT is an emergency and should be evaluated and treated by a qualified physician. The faster interventions are started, the less inflammation and damage will be sustained.

60: PROMOTES URINARY HEALTH

Urinary tract infection (UTI) describes acute, common urinary problems caused by pathogens in the urinary bladder, the urethra, ureters, and even kidneys. There is a spectrum of infection that ranges from simple dysbiosis (a disruption in the urinary microbiome) to inflammatory infection.

UTIs are characterized by an urgency to urinate, frequent urination, and burning. Adult women used to be the main sufferers of UTIs, but more and more children with normal urinary tract structure and function are experiencing them.

Many pathogens have the ability to move about. It is hypothesized that pathogens from the vaginal and/or intestinal tracts enter the urinary system and establish residence, causing an imbalance in the resident microbiome. That is one reason why wiping from front to back when using the bathroom and urinating after sex are important UTI preventative measures.

Nearly all UTIs are treated with antibiotics, but this has consequences. It was believed in the past that the urinary bladder was sterile, and thus urine was sterile. Recent advances in microbial identification methods show that the bladder, urinary tract, and urine are not sterile, and in fact are home to a community of microbes not yet characterized. As a result, recklessly killing suspected pathogens with antibiotics may disrupt the resident urinary microbiome, just as it disrupts the gastrointestinal microbiome, setting the stage for increased dysbiosis.

Instead of antibiotics for UTI preventive treatments, oral probiotics are now being investigated. Many *Lactobacillus* species have antagonistic activities against common urinary pathogens, and may be recommended prophylactic treatments in the future. As of now, no blanket recommendations are embraced. However, probiotics in general can promote urinary health. They protect against pathogens in the GI tract and vagina that can migrate to the urinary tract, and protect against the deleterious effects of antibiotics.

61: LIMITS YEAST INFECTIONS

Have you ever baked bread and had to proof the yeast? Proofing the yeast allows it to become active in the conditions it prefers the most: warm and moist with access to sugar. Baker's and brewer's yeast are both forms of *Saccharomyces* yeasts, as is *Saccharomyces boulardii,* but these yeasts are usually helpful to you and noninfectious, except in immunocompromised people or people with yeast allergies.

Candida yeast species, on the other hand, can cause numerous infections in and on you. Although they are usually present in controlled amounts, *Candida* overcomes your usual defenses and establishes itself when conditions are favorable, such as when you take antibiotics and many beneficial bacteria, which normally would control *Candida*, are killed. Unlike the *Saccharomyces* yeasts, which are not invasive, *Candida* species form *hyphae,* finger-like projections that penetrate tissues, causing deep infections that are difficult to eliminate. *Candida* is also able to weaken your immune defenses.

Candida albicans is the most common species that causes yeast infections, but there are others. It is a normal inhabitant of the gastrointestinal tract and is often found in the female vaginal tract. *Candida* infections on the skin cause red, itchy rashes that often weep moisture, and in the vagina there is often a cottage-cheese-like discharge in addition to the skin symptoms.

The conventional treatment for *Candida* infections is antifungal medication. However, just as bacteria are becoming resistant to antibiotics, *Candida* is becoming resistant to antifungals. Numerous probiotics have antagonistic actions against *Candida*, but once it is established, it may take combination therapies to control it.

Keeping gut microbiota balanced with probiotics will help prevent or limit *Candida* infections, regardless of where they appear. If you have recurrent yeast infections, please have the *Candida* species identified by a specialist so that the correct antifungals, proper diet, and probiotics can be prescribed.

62: IMPROVES ALZHEIMER'S DISEASE

Alzheimer's disease (AD) is a common form of senile dementia. The cognitive impairments begin with short-term memory loss and progress until a person loses his or her sense of self. Oxidative stress, which is an imbalance between free-radical production and antioxidant status, and inflammation, including neuroinflammation, are common in AD. These result in the death of neuronal connections and neurons in the brain with overall shrinkage of the brain.

Although the exact causes of AD are unknown, insulin resistance, hyperglycemia, and dysregulation of blood lipids are associated with the initiation and progression of the disease. Genetics, environmental causes, and lifestyle factors most likely also play a role.

Since probiotics are known to benefit other mental and emotional conditions, researchers are investigating probiotics in terms of AD. So far the results are promising. AD patients who received a probiotic supplement containing *Lactobacillus acidophilus, casei* and *fermentum*, and *Bifidobacterium bifidum*, showed a significant improvement in mental state evaluation, with decreases in markers of oxidative stress,

inflammation, insulin resistance, lipids, and others.

Probiotics may be an upcoming therapy for AD, but you don't have to wait until symptoms of AD appear before taking action. As mentioned previously, probiotics work best as preventive agents, preventing detrimental changes to the digestive, immune, endocrine, and nervous (including brain) systems, as well as other body systems. Since your gastrointestinal tract is the main site of probiotic actions, keeping yours balanced with probiotics of many kinds may be an unrecognized way to thwart the development or severity of AD.

63: REDUCES CAUSES OF ANXIETY

Anxiety is a normal reaction to situations that are unfamiliar, and it brings with it a heightened sense of stress. While occasional anxiety is normal, anxiety becomes a disorder when it is persistent, overwhelming, and interferes with everyday activities.

There are many types of anxiety disorders, such as generalized anxiety disorder (GAD), panic disorder, social anxiety disorder, and separation anxiety, but what they all have in common is that they seem to be uncontrollable. It can seem like no matter how much you try to rationalize with your brain that you are overreacting, the effort is futile.

The gut microbiome is known to affect cognitive functions such as anxiety. Studies show that introducing a pathogen in low doses in animals can create anxiety even without an immune response to the pathogen or an established infection. Studies also show that taking the feces from an anxious rodent and transplanting them into a non-anxious rodent causes the nonanxious rodent to develop anxiety.

Probiotics of many types can help with anxiety by controlling the pathogens that induce anxiety, and by interacting with the enteric nervous system in the gut as well as the vagal nerve, which runs from the brain to the abdomen and gastrointestinal tract. Also, probiotics, particularly many *Lactobacillus* and *Bifidobacterium* species, produce neurotransmitters that interact with your own neurotransmitters to produce a calming effect to reduce levels of stress that contribute to anxiety.

Anxiety is a normal response to unfamiliar situations, but it can become crippling and persistent. Probiotics work on some of the root causes of anxiety without the side effects of drugs such as benzodiazepines.

DON'T STOP YOUR PRESCRIPTION MEDICATIONS

If you are being treated for anxiety with medications, do not abruptly stop taking your medications. Doing so could have serious mental and physical consequences.

64: MAY HELP WITH BIPOLAR DISEASE

Bipolar disease (BD), also known as manic-depressive illness, is a mental disorder characterized by extreme changes in mood, energy, and activity levels. These changes fall along a spectrum of subtypes, with depressive episodes and manic episodes having varying lengths of time and intensity, so BD may be different among individuals.

Risk factors are unclear, but decreases in brain volume, alterations in brain structure, altered brain functioning, and family history/genetics seem to be associated with BD. Conventional treatment consists of psychotherapy and psychiatric medications such as mood stabilizers, antipsychotics, and antidepressants.

Investigations into the role of the gut microbiome in BD have only recently been initiated, but preliminary findings from stool analysis show that there is dysbiosis, a disruption in the gut microbiome, in patients with BD. They also show that the ratio of pro-inflammatory molecules to anti-inflammatory molecules is tipped toward inflammation, that there is immune dysregulation, and that there is an increased immune response to yeast.

Probiotics of many types may help with BD by controlling the influence of pathogens and the relative proportions of microbes within the gastrointestinal tract in dysbiosis. By doing so, they will also decrease pro-inflammatory molecules within and away from the gut. Probiotics can have anti-inflammatory actions and balance the immune response for a more appropriate reaction. Although many probiotics can do these things, any *Saccharomyces* should not be used unless tests that are run to determine immune sensitivity to them do not detect an immune reaction.

CAUTION: DON'T STOP MEDS

Do not abruptly stop taking any psychiatric medications, as doing so can result in worsening of symptoms and uncomfortable and/or dangerous withdrawal reactions. Please consult your mental health professional with questions.

65: CLEARS BRAIN FOG

Do you ever feel like your thinking is clouded, where it is hard to think, hard to focus, and hard to recall events that happened recently? You may have a case of brain fog. Brain fog is a group of neurocognitive symptoms that make a person feel groggy and not quite "with it." There are many causes, such as lack of sleep, a hangover, fever and illness, neurotoxins such as MSG, chronic inflammation, infections, autoimmune disease, heavy metals toxicity, consumption of reactive foods, vitamin deficiencies, blood sugar fluctuations, hormonal fluctuations, and bacterial by-products. The end result is neuroinflammation, which causes the clouded thinking.

When looking at the list of possible causes, it is no surprise that gut function plays a role in brain fog. The gastrointestinal (GI) tract is in direct and indirect communication with the brain, and microbes in the gut can affect, for better or for worse, the types of communication that occur between the GI tract and the brain. Additionally, harmful products from pathogens in the gut can travel to the liver, overloading the liver and causing toxins to be circulated to the brain and contributing to brain fog.

Probiotics can play a major positive role in brain fog. *Lactobacillus*, in particular, can produce neurotransmitters used for brain neuron-to-neuron transmission to facilitate thinking. Probiotics can interact with the vagus nerve to the brain, with the enteric nervous system that can communicate with the brain, and with the brain via chemical messengers.

Probiotics in general can also balance immune function, influence hormone levels, aid in digestion and nutrient absorption, produce some vitamins, and balance blood sugar insulin responses. By preventing and reducing leaky gut and controlling levels of pathogens, probiotics reduce harmful bacterial by-products that can enter the brain and contribute to brain fog.

66: ALLEVIATES DEPRESSION

Everyone has their ups and downs, but how resilient you are to the downs can determine if you develop depression. Depression has many levels of severity, from mild to moderate to severe, and an estimated 350 million people worldwide suffer from it.

Depression often goes hand in hand with anxiety. Both conditions can have origins in the gastrointestinal (GI) tract, which typical antidepressants and benzodiazepine medications do not address. Since there is a connection between the health of the GI tract and the health of the nervous system/brain, directly through the vagus nerve and also via indirect chemical effects, improving the former can positively affect the latter.

Improving the health of your GI tract involves removing foods, drinks, and toxins that are irritating to it and your nervous, immune, and endocrine systems. It also involves finding out what nutrients and substances you are low in or missing, and reinoculating with beneficial microbes such as probiotics.

Many *Lactobacillus* and *Bifidobacterium* species are naturals at protecting and improving gut health. Additionally, research in animals and humans has shown that probiotics decrease scores on depression assessments, thereby alleviating depression. As a matter of fact, there is a new term, *psychobiotics*, for these microbes that influence mental health conditions like depression.

Cleaning up your diet to remove things that bother you and to add nutrients you and your microbiota need, physical activity to reduce stress and increase feel-good neurotransmitters, mindfulness to discover how your thoughts affect your feelings, and daily consumption of probiotics are easy ways to improve your mental health outlook.

SEEK APPROPRIATE HELP

If you think you are suffering from depression, please seek appropriate help. Probiotics can help with the causes of symptoms in some depressed states, but should not be a replacement for care from a qualified health professional.

67: ADDRESSES HEADACHES

What causes your headaches? You may know what usually triggers yours, but there can be many, many causes of headaches. Defining the cause has to take into account the type of headache: Is it primary, as in a tension, migraine, or cluster headache? Or is the headache secondary to, say, sinus pressure, a hangover, or a rebound headache caused by frequently taking headache medications so that when you don't, you actually get a headache from persistent pain? Or is it from nerve or facial pain?

As with other health conditions, the best thing to do regarding headaches is to try to prevent them. One of the sites for the primary origin of your headache could be your GI tract. Medications like aspirin, acetaminophen, ibuprofen, and naproxen sodium may relieve your headache, but they are taxing to the liver and gastrointestinal (GI) tract and could be adding to the problem.

Probiotics of many types can be part of your preventative therapy for headaches since they provide benefits for the disruptions in your GI tract that could be causing your headaches. Toxins from pathogens can leave the GI tract and sensitize cells that contribute to headaches, so pathogen control is one way probiotics can help. Additionally, assistance with digestion, absorption, and motility, and balancing the immune response in the face of food allergies or sensitivities, are other ways that probiotics can reduce the disturbances in the GI tract that contribute to headaches.

68: IMPROVES HEPATIC ENCEPHALOPATHY

Hepatic encephalopathy (HE) is a condition in which the liver is too overloaded to properly remove toxins from the blood, resulting in brain function problems. There is a spectrum of HE, with mild forms (minimal HE) exhibiting brain fog–like memory, disorientation, and concentration problems. The most severe forms can result in coma and death. HE can also be acute or chronic. HE is most frequently seen in liver cirrhosis, in which the liver is scarred and unable to function.

There are several theories regarding the origin of HE. One is that specialized cells in the brain, astrocytes, experience structural and functional changes, thereby reducing their effectiveness. Astrocytes contribute to the protection of the brain by detoxifying toxins, such as ammonia, in the blood before they cross the blood-brain barrier and enter the brain. Ammonia is considered an important player in HE because it is very toxic to the brain, causing increased oxidative stress.

Although ammonia can be produced in many tissues, the greatest source is the gastrointestinal (GI) tract. Two conventional protocols for prevention and treatment of HE consist of a minimally absorbed antibiotic, such as rifaximin, to kill bacteria that contribute to ammonia production, or lactulose to encourage the growth of beneficial bacteria such as *Lactobacillus*. Discontinuation of the treatments results in high relapse rates.

Probiotics taken consistently may provide preventative as well as therapeutic benefits for HE. Probiotics can control the populations of bacteria contributing to excess ammonia production, produce short-chain fatty acids to lower intestinal pH, decrease intestinal permeability, and decrease inflammatory and oxidative stress molecules that can damage the liver and brain.

69: SOOTHES IRRITABILITY

Irritability is a feeling of agitation, a mood in which you are upset or frustrated easily. You may feel loss of control. It could have psychological causes, such as stress perception, anxiety, depression, or other mental health conditions, or it could be caused by physical things, such as being too hot/cold, being sleep deprived, illness, pain, low blood sugar, hormone fluctuations, or addiction withdrawal. It could also be a combination of several things that when added together push past your internal capacity of patience. In its basic form, irritability is a collection of stressors.

Other sections in this book show how the health of your gastrointestinal (GI) microbiome and probiotics are involved with many of the psychological and physical stressors previously listed that are involved with irritability, so please read those sections and look at the health of your GI tract.

The collection of stressors that contribute to irritability result in stress on your body. Probiotics, such as *Lactobacillus* and *Bifidobacterium* species, can help produce small amounts of B vitamins to help you deal with stress. They can also reduce pathogens that produce substances that could be clouding your thinking and attenuate the neurotransmitters and hormones involved in your stress response.

In many cases you can choose to be irritable—by not dealing with relationships and letting things bother you—or not. Reducing the triggers, including those caused by problems in the gut, with probiotics could make irritability a thing of the past.

TO MAKE A SNACK TO CURB IRRITABILITY, USE

This snack provides protein, fats, probiotics, B vitamins, magnesium, and other nutrients to help you feel less irritable.

½ cup plain organic Greek yogurt that has extra probiotics added

2 tablespoons sliced almonds or chopped walnuts

½ cup raspberries and/or blueberries

Layer the ingredients in a bowl and enjoy!

70: MAY HELP SCHIZOPHRENIA

Schizophrenia is a severe and chronic mental disorder that may make those afflicted feel like their reality is distorted. Some sufferers have hallucinations, delusions, and/or thought and movement disorders during positive symptoms, and hyporeactions to emotions and behavior during negative symptoms. Other symptoms may be cognitive in nature, with limited ability to understand information, limited ability to focus, and problems with working memory.

The exact cause of schizophrenia is unknown, but suspected factors are interactions between genes and the environment, and different brain structure and chemical and neurotransmitter reactions in the brain. Symptoms usually begin between the ages of sixteen and thirty.

Although the exact cause of schizophrenia is not known, research shows that schizophrenia is associated with inflammatory and immune responses. The sources of these responses are believed to be dysfunctions in the brain-gut axis, hypersensitivity to food antigens (particularly gluten and cow's milk casein), hypersensitivity to yeast, gut permeability, and dysbiosis (a disruption of the normal gut microbiota).

Probiotics of many types may help schizophrenia in several ways: by controlling the relative proportions of microbes within the gastrointestinal tract, and particularly pathogens in dysbiosis; by preventing gut permeability; by decreasing pro-inflammatory molecules within and away from the gut; by balancing the immune response with potential anti-inflammatory actions for a more appropriate response; and by improving digestion and nutrient absorption. Although many probiotics can do these things, any *Saccharomyces* should not be used unless tests show that there is no immune sensitivity to them.

PROBIOTICS ARE NOT A SUBSTITUTE FOR YOUR PSYCHIATRIC MEDS

Do not abruptly stop taking any psychiatric medications, as doing so can result in worsening of symptoms and uncomfortable and/or dangerous withdrawal reactions. Please consult your mental health professional if you wish to wean off medications.

71: REDUCES SUGAR CRAVINGS

You experience that afternoon slump and reach for a candy bar or a sugar-laden coffee. Or maybe you go through your day, starting with a breakfast of doughnuts or sugary cereal, and then proceed to sodas for drinks, cookies to snack on, dessert after dinner, and finally to a nighttime snack of ice cream. You know that feeling; it's that I-have-to-have-something-sweet-and-I-have-to-have-it-NOW feeling.

Sugar is so easily accessible in Westernized cultures that it is easy to overindulge in it. But why do you crave it? There are several reasons. One, sugar usually means sucrose, which is composed of glucose and fructose. Glucose is the sugar in your blood, so consumption of sugar results in a temporary boost of energy. However, that blood-sugar spike causes insulin to be released to usher the sugar into cells for energy or fat storage, and shortly afterward your blood sugar drops. So then you feel a slump and reach for something to bring your blood sugar back up: more sugar.

Another reason is that sugar is addictive. Sugar intake causes the release of dopamine, a feel-good neurotransmitter involved in motivation, reward, and reinforcement of pleasurable behavior in your brain, similar to what other drugs of abuse do. As a result, you crave that good feeling and so indulge regularly in sugar.

Another reason may be that your gut microbiota influences your behavior. Pathogens, in particular, are able to use sucrose to outpace the growth of beneficial microbes and thus can affect brain function with their metabolites. Some pathogens produce by-products of sugar metabolism that may promote addiction.

Many probiotics can help control pathogens, regulate hormones involved in appetite, influence neurotransmitter actions and production, and modulate insulin release. With the help of probiotics, you may be able to kick your sugar addiction!

72: MINIMIZES ACNE

Acne can affect adolescents as well as adults. Acne is usually blamed on three factors: overproduction of the protective oil in the skin, irregular shedding of dead skin cells, and/or buildup of bacteria.

There are many causes for these three factors, including diet, hormone imbalances, genetics, and topical application of pore-clogging or oil-stripping personal-care products. A diet filled with processed and high-sugar foods is more inflammatory and contributes to inflammation in the skin. This type of diet also preferentially benefits pathogens in the gastrointestinal tract that contribute to inflammation and hormonal imbalances. So, acne has a link with what is going on inside your body, and probiotics can benefit you there. In fact, there are a few probiotic products, containing *Lactobacillus* and *Bifidobacterium* species, taken internally that are marketed to help with acne.

Acne is also linked to conditions in your skin itself. Your skin has its own microbiome, and different species of microbes prefer different environments. By using harsh acne products, antibacterial products, and products with oil-stripping ingredients such as sodium laurel sulfate on your skin, you are disrupting the eco-balance on your skin.

Topically applied probiotics can benefit acne. Even if the species used are not the same as the species that normally would have inhabited your face, chest, or back, the probiotics can have beneficial actions such as producing acidic and antimicrobial products to control the growth of skin-inflaming microbes, interacting with your skin to improve its defenses, and controlling pH so that your skin functions normally and keeps its barrier more intact. There are several topical probiotic products on the market that may accomplish those things.

While your first reaction to acne may be to bombard it with an arsenal of harsh products, a gentler approach, from the inside as well as the outside, may be a better option.

73: REDUCES AGING FROM SUN EXPOSURE

Long, lazy days at the beach seem like the ultimate way to relax. Images of suntanned bodies and sun-streaked hair have the ultimate sex appeal for many people. Sunshine can make you feel awake and energetic. While some sun exposure is indeed beneficial and necessary, over time all of that sun exposure can take a toll on your skin and accelerate its aging.

Sun-parched skin can be dry, thickened, and wrinkly. Even routine tanning can lead to those effects. Too much sun exposure can also cause skin cancers in susceptible folks.

While it is always a good idea to practice safe sun exposure by covering up exposed areas after short exposure and using nontoxic sunscreens, there is a way to help protect against the aging effects of sun exposure from the inside out and the outside in with probiotics.

Numerous probiotics, such as the *Lactobacillus* and *Bifidobacterium* species, taken internally can help suppress water loss from the skin, improve plumpness of the skin, reduce thickening, and improve skin elasticity. One way they do this is by regulating the immune system to suppress inflammatory chemicals from attacking collagen, structure of the skin, and detoxification organs such as the liver. They can also make skin-friendly nutrients more available to your body and reduce pathogenic bacteria in your digestive tract that contribute to inflammation in your body.

Applied topically, experiments showed that probiotics can provide antioxidant protection to the skin to help guard against free-radical damage and also help maintain a normal skin barrier.

If you want to reduce aging from sun exposure, practice smart sun exposure and nourish your skin topically and from the inside out with probiotics!

74: FIGHTS ATHLETE'S FOOT

Athlete's foot, or *tinea pedis*, is a contagious fungal infection that affects the skin on the feet. It can occur on the soles, toe webs, or anywhere else on the feet. Usual symptoms of the most common type of athlete's foot are itchy and cracked skin, stinging, rawness, and moist, white, scaly lesions. Another type of athlete's foot is a dry scaly form that causes redness in a moccasin-like area over the soles of the feet.

The fungus that causes athlete's foot can be found on floors and clothing. That is why it is a good idea to wear sandals in communal showers and locker rooms, wear your own socks and shoes, rotate shoes to allow them to dry out, and wash socks in hot water. The fungus requires a warm, dark, and humid environment in order to grow, so keeping the feet aired and dry and changing socks frequently is a must if you have athlete's foot.

Athlete's foot is usually not a serious health concern, but if you have diabetes or are otherwise immunocompromised, it can progress to more serious issues. The skin microbiome and barrier are disrupted in athlete's foot, setting the stage for secondary bacterial infection to develop. If the redness becomes more painful and more widespread and/or deep, those could be signs that a bacterial infection has established itself.

Athlete's foot is usually treated with over-the-counter antifungal medications, but it is important to follow directions carefully so that the fungus does not develop resistance to the product. Probiotics taken internally can help with athlete's foot by improving your skin's barrier protection, maintaining adequate skin moisture, and reducing inflammation. Topical application of probiotics may benefit athlete's foot because many probiotics have antifungal actions.

75: BATTLES BAD BREATH

Bad breath, also called halitosis, can be caused by odorous foods such as garlic, onions, strong cheeses, coffee, and alcoholic drinks. It can also be caused by conditions such as burping, reflux, sinus infections, and postnasal drip, or even by more serious conditions, but in many cases it is caused by an upset in the microbial balance in your mouth.

When you eat, microbes in your mouth start feasting on the food, mucus, and shed cells in your mouth. If you have an imbalance of microbes, with pathogens such as *Fusobacterium* and *Porphyromonas* present in uncontrolled amounts, those microbes can produce hydrogen sulfide and mercaptan, two smelly substances. Most people equate hydrogen sulfide to the smell of rotten eggs.

Since bad breath is primarily a result of dysbiosis, an imbalance of microbes in the mouth and digestive tract, probiotics are a natural choice as a remedy. Probiotics can help you digest food so that you are less likely to burp up nasty smells. They also are able to control pathogens that release the smelly sulfuric compounds in your mouth. Taken internally, probiotics, and especially lactic acid bacteria such as *Lactobacillus* species and *Weissella*

cibaria, can resolve the root causes of your bad breath so you can walk out the door without breath mints.

76: REDUCES BELCHING AND BURPING

Belching, more commonly known as burping, is a forced expulsion of gas from the stomach. The air or gas causes uncomfortable symptoms by producing stomach distension. Not only is the sound embarrassing in most cultures, but the gas can have the smell of the mix of food consumed.

Many times the gas is swallowed air caused by smoking, talking while eating, eating too quickly, mindlessly swallowing, chewing gum, gulping drinks, or drinking while eating. Other times carbonated drinks or beer can cause burping. Sometimes the cause is an underlying condition, such as heartburn or inflammation of the stomach, as with ulcers.

Other times the reason for your belching may be indigestion. Foods that are not properly digested can lead to excess fermentation or putrefaction, with increased gas production as a result. Foods that are not properly moved along the gastrointestinal tract, due to problems with motility, can have the same consequences.

Probiotics of many types may be able to help reduce your burping. Probiotics can improve digestion, and can help normalize the nerve and muscle functions of the intestines to improve motility. While it is always good eating etiquette to chew thoroughly, not talk with food in your mouth, not drink to wash food down your esophagus (unless it is stuck, of course), and not gulp down drinks, oral probiotics can provide another way to reduce the chances of excess and exaggerated burping.

77: MINIMIZES BLOATING

The waistband of your pants feels tight and your abdomen feels like an inflated balloon. You may be burping and passing gas. You are probably experiencing bloating. One of the most common causes of bloating is overeating. The next time you eat, slow down and chew. Try also eating smaller portions of food.

Other common causes of bloating include:

- Swallowing too much air while eating
- Not properly digesting foods
- Not moving those foods along the digestive tract
- Having an imbalance of gut microbes

Many foods that are nutritious for you can cause excess gas production in your intestines. Foods such as beans, and cruciferous vegetables such as asparagus, cabbage, and cauliflower, contain healthy fiber, but if your gut microbiota are not in the correct proportions or are not accustomed to those types of fiber, they could have a fermentation party and produce excess gas. If the time it takes for food to move through your digestive tract is too slow, you could be allowing excess gas to form. Often, a disruption in the ratio of helpful to harmful microbes in your digestive tract is the cause of your bloating.

Conventional treatment for bloating is over-the-counter gas medication containing simethicone, the same medication commonly given to infants with colic. This medication does not treat the causes of your bloating, just your symptoms.

Probiotics of many types can help address the causes of bloating. They assist with the digestion and absorption of foods and the movement of food through your gastrointestinal tract so that it does not stagnate. They also correct a disruption in gut microbiota. Use probiotics regularly to target the causes and minimize bloating!

78: LESSENS SWEATY BODY ODOR

We have all been in a situation in which we suddenly realize that we smell stinky. While movement, stress, hygiene, diet, and multiple other factors can contribute to the intensity of the odor, the blame for the creation of much of that smell belongs to the bacteria that inhabit your underarms.

You have between 3 and 4 million sweat glands over most of your body to regulate body temperature and remove toxins and wastes. Some of the sweat glands, like those in your armpits, respond to stress.

Current research shows that non-probiotic bacteria, *Corynebacterium* and *Staphylococcus*, in particular, feed on sweat and generate underarm odor. While these bacteria are normal inhabitants of your body, their numbers can increase when conditions favor their growth, resulting in more stench. The key to reducing the odor is to keep these bacteria numbers low.

Most people try to control these bacterial numbers by using antiperspirants to prevent underarm sweating or by trying to kill microbes with anti-perspirant or antimicrobial products. Research shows that in addition to being harmful to the body, those methods may actually increase the number of odor generators. However, keeping the underarm at its preferred low pH can control them.

Probiotics that are aerotolerant, such as many *Lactobacillus* and *Bacillus coagulans* or *subtilis*, are used in many commercial probiotic deodorant recipes. These bacteria can help maintain a low pH while letting the body sweat to remove toxins and wastes. Additionally, eating real food and taking food, drink, or supplement sources of probiotics can change the composition of sweat to be less odoriferous.

A RECIPE TO BEAT ODOR

A simple recipe to try to jump-start a balanced skin microbiome is to mix a capsule of a shelf-stable probiotic containing *Lactobacillus* and/or *Bacillus* with a starch such as potato starch. Add water to make a thin paste and apply to clean underarms. Store any extra in refrigerator. Exact proportions will vary depending on skin sensitivity and odor level.

79: IMPROVES FISHY BODY ODOR

Trimethylaminuria (TMAU) is a condition in which a person has a fishy body odor. It is a medical metabolic condition that has little to do with levels of hygiene. In TMAU, the liver cannot break down an odorous substance called TMA into a nonodorous substance, either due to genetics (primary TMAU) or due to a problem in organs of elimination, stress, hormone fluctuations, or dietary overload of foods containing TMA or TMAO (secondary TMAU). The TMA is then released in sweat, urine, reproductive fluids, and breath. Since humans perspire throughout the day, even unnoticeably, the odor reappears even with frequent showering.

TMA is found in products such as red meats, energy supplements, eggs, liver, soybeans, marine life, mustard, whole grains, legumes, cruciferous vegetables, beets, processed cereals, some greens and some beans, as well as a multitude of other foods. You can see that trying to restrict all sources of TMA would result in a restricted diet and possible lack of nutrients.

If you have a fishy body smell, you should see a doctor to determine the cause so that undetected organ problems do not go undiagnosed.

Conditions such as fatty liver are common causes of secondary TMAU.

Probiotics taken daily help with TMAU by improving the function of organs of elimination, such as the intestines, liver, kidneys, skin, and lungs. They can also control populations of pathogens that can release TMA from foods, thus reducing the body's burden of TMA.

TMAU IS A DIFFICULT CONDITION TO LIVE WITH

Remember, a person with fishy body odor does not necessarily have poor hygiene. He may have primary or secondary TMAU, and along with dietary help and probiotic intake, he needs understanding from loved ones, coworkers, and the public.

80: FIGHTS CAVITIES

The shrill sound of a dentist's drill on cavities can cause stress. It is important to drill out the decayed part of the tooth before filling it, however, to remove bacteria that may be hiding in it. But what causes cavities?

The World Health Organization states that dental cavities are found worldwide in 60–90 percent of school-age children and nearly 100 percent of adults. Cavities are caused by a breakdown in tooth enamel that occurs when acids eat away at the enamel, exposing the softer dentin beneath. While acidic foods and drinks (such as sodas and sugary lemonade) can dissolve enamel, a common culprit of acid production in the mouth is bacteria.

One of the pathogenic bacteria associated with cavities is *Streptococcus mutans*, though there are others. *S. mutans* forms a biofilm called plaque with other microbes that allows a safe haven for the microbes to flourish. *S. mutans* takes sugars and simple carbohydrates (think most breads, crackers, pretzels, baked goods, and so on) you eat and uses them as fuel while producing acids.

Probiotics can help reduce the numbers of *S. mutans* in the mouth, even if the probiotics are dead, thus reducing plaque, acid production, and the potential for cavities. Reducing the types of foods that fuel the bacteria that contribute to cavities, practicing proper oral hygiene, and adding probiotics and fermented foods and drinks containing probiotic-like microbes can make the sound of a dentist's drill a thing of the past.

81: DIMINISHES COLD SORES

Cold sores, sometimes called fever blisters, are clusters of small blisters usually found around the lip area. When they break open, a crust forms over the sore until it heals. They can be itchy, tingly, painful, and make you self-conscious.

Cold sores are neither caused by colds nor by fevers, but instead are caused by an oral herpes virus, usually herpes simplex virus 1 (HSV-1). The virus is spread through close contact with someone, such as kissing, sharing drinks and utensils, and sharing personal products such as towels. Many people are carriers of the virus and never have outbreaks, but for those that do, outbreaks typically happen in the same places. This is because the virus lies dormant in nerve cells until it seizes an opportunity to reactivate. Viruses like HSV-1 are tenacious and usually stay in the body for life.

Conventional treatment involves skin creams or ointments and antiviral medications. In most cases, no treatment is necessary as the sore will heal with time. One way to diminish cold sores may be with probiotics. Since the HSV-1 virus lies dormant and can reactivate, the key to keeping it dormant is to keep your immune system balanced and able to suppress it. Probiotics are very good at modulating the immune system so that it can deal with invaders such as viruses and pathogenic bacteria. Taken orally, probiotics interact with your immune system in your intestines as well as with remote immune protectors.

Probiotics can also help you digest foods and absorb nutrients, such as vitamins A, C, and E, and minerals such as zinc, which support your immune system. Get to the root cause of your cold sores with probiotics!

82: LESSENS DANDRUFF

Dandruff can make a person self-conscious. Dandruff symptoms are white, oily-looking flakes of dead skin that can clump together or independently flake off. Sometimes the scalp is itchy and scaly looking.

The most common conventional treatment for dandruff is a special shampoo containing pyrithione zinc, a complex of zinc with the ability to inhibit bacterial and fungal proliferation. Unfortunately, those shampoos also contain the very ingredient, sodium laurel (laureth) sulfate, that strips the scalp skin of its natural protective barrier and protective microbiota.

The most commonly touted causes of dandruff are red, irritated oily skin, overly dry scalp skin, or yeast colonization. What they all have in common, however, is that the scalp skin barrier is compromised by a disruption in the normal microbiota. This disruption can happen from changes on the outside of the skin as well as on the inside, so treating one side without treating the other may be a waste of time.

Probiotics can lessen dandruff from the inside by supporting the skin barrier, but skin-irritating products should be discontinued. By increasing skin moisture and resiliency, oral probiotics can help the scalp produce proper levels of antimicrobials and oils to control microbe populations and protect the skin. Oral probiotics can also aid in the absorption of nutrients needed for skin health.

TO MAKE A RINSE TO LESSEN DANDRUFF, FOLLOW THESE INSTRUCTIONS

While not studied in research as of yet, adding yogurt or kefir to your scalp may help to lessen dandruff by reducing scalp pH, adding moisture, and helping support the normal inhabitants of the scalp.

Here is what you need: Plain, real yogurt or kefir cultured from milk with no added ingredients (enough to thinly spread on your scalp).

Apply yogurt or kefir to your scalp for 20 minutes and then rinse out. Avoid using harsh shampoos. Repeat the treatment two to three times per week and then taper off to a maintenance routine.

83: RELIEVES ECZEMA

Flare-ups of itchy, red, scaly, dry, and cracked skin with possible blisters on the face, hands, feet, inner elbows, or back of knees is usually diagnosed as eczema. Eczema is a chronic inflammatory condition of the skin that often begins in infancy. It is more common in Westernized societies, affects more than half of newborns during their first year of life, affects one-third of infants, and may afflict adults. Eighty percent of children with eczema will develop seasonal allergies or asthma within five years. Thus, prevention can save a lot of suffering in both children and adults.

Exact causes of eczema are unknown, but there is a loss of skin barrier integrity, which allows moisture to escape and microbes to enter. Scratching can cause infections requiring antibiotics. Conventional treatments such as moisturizing creams, steroid creams and ointments, immune-regulating drugs, and ultraviolet light aim to suppress symptoms, but do not address the underlying cause of immune dysfunction.

Eczema itself may or may not be a true allergic reaction, but in either case, a disruption in the gut microbiome with immune system involvement is present. Probiotics are a natural choice for imbalances in both the gut microbiome and the immune system in eczema since the correct probiotics can help tip both imbalances back to more balanced states. Probiotics can also improve the skin barrier, helping with hydration and lessening irritation.

Success with probiotics for eczema occurs more frequently when started in pregnant mothers and in infants at risk of eczema. Improvement of the vaginal environment, of the microbial composition of mothers' breast milks, and in the infants' developing immune systems are all probiotic actions. Nonetheless, probiotics may help with eczema in adults too.

84: WHITENS EYES

When you look at a person's face, one of the first things you notice is his or her eyes. Someone with eyes that look awake and engaged with the world, with bright whites and a spark to them, is more attractive than someone whose eyes are half-closed, dull-looking, or have a yellowish tint to the whites.

It is often said that the eyes are the windows to the soul, but they can also be a window into the status of someone's health. For example, someone with red, bloodshot eyes may have dry eyes, allergies, pink eye, tired eyes from working at a computer or lack of sleep, may have indulged in alcohol or other drugs, or may be ill. But what about when the whites of the eyes are yellowish?

Yellowing of the whites of the eyes is usually caused by jaundice. Jaundice reflects a problem with too many red blood cells being broken down and/or an overburdened liver. Your liver dismantles old red blood cells, and one component, bilirubin, should be filtered out of the blood and secreted in bile to be eliminated in stool. Any problem with the liver or bile ducts can cause bilirubin to back up into the blood and cause yellowing of the whites of the eyes and skin.

Oral probiotics alleviate jaundice by reducing the amount of intestinal toxins that go from the intestines to the liver, and by keeping the bowels moving so that wastes are eliminated in a timely manner. It is up to you to be awake and engaged with the world in order to have sparkly, captivating eyes, but probiotics taken daily can help you keep the whites of your eyes a brighter white!

85: REDUCES SMELLY GAS

Everyone passes gas. Most people pass it twenty times per day or less, and while it may have a slight odor, it should not smell like a dark green cloud of toxic fumes. If it does, you probably have some kind of gastrointestinal (GI) problem going on.

Most people try to treat the symptoms of flatulence with medications such as simethicone without targeting the causes based on what is happening in the digestive tract. It is normal to swallow air while talking, eating, eating too quickly, mindlessly swallowing, chewing gum, gulping drinks, or drinking while eating. It is also normal to get gas in your GI tract from carbonated drinks or from normal digestion, particularly from fiber-containing foods. However, routinely having gas from indigestion, constipation, diarrhea, and GI disorders is not normal.

Many bacteria and yeasts in your GI tract release gases when they break down the foods you eat. These gases are not smelly, but other trace gases, such as sulfur-based ones, are. Probiotics can speed up or provide missing microbes for the turnover of your microbiota to microbes that can utilize the fibers and other compounds in nutritious foods. Probiotics can also help you digest foods better and regulate elimination of wastes, so that undigested foods are not putrefying in your digestive tract.

Unless contraindicated by your doctor, eating high-fiber and high-sulfur foods is excellent for your health. If you avoid only the items you know you cannot digest, such as milk products if you are lactose intolerant, you can eat a healthy diet and not have putrid-smelling gas with the help of probiotics!

86: FIGHTS BLEEDING GUMS

An attractive smile can help you feel good about yourself, so you brush, floss, and use mouthwash religiously in the hopes that your mouth will look fresh and clean. However, you can still end up with puffy, bleeding gums in a condition called gingivitis.

Gingivitis is a mild form of periodontal disease that is limited to the part of your gums at the base of your teeth. Bacteria and yeasts in your mouth coexist with saliva and other substances in your mouth and form protective biofilms, colonies of different microbes that survive by sharing resources. Plaque is a form of biofilm, so it is necessary to brush your teeth in order to remove it. If plaque stays undisturbed, it forms tartar, which then requires professional cleaning to remove. Plaque and tartar buildup are the perfect environments for pathogenic bacteria that cause gum diseases to flourish.

Brushing your teeth gently, so as not to tear your gums, and flossing regularly are easy ways to prevent gingivitis. You may think that using a harsh mouthwash containing alcohol is necessary to control the bacteria that cause gum disease, but that is not true. Harsh mouthwash will temporarily kill many bacteria on the surfaces of your mouth and teeth, but it also dries out your mouth, and the reservoir of microbes at your gum line will soon proliferate again. The way to control the disease-causing bacteria is through competitiveness with helpful bacteria such as probiotics.

Probiotics can bind to pathogens, stop them from adhering to your gums and forming plaque, crowd them out, and even disable them. They also help balance your immune system so that immune responses to pathogens are appropriate, but not excessive. Probiotics taken daily can fight bleeding gums at the source.

87: LESSENS HAIR LOSS

Hair loss has many causes. Some of the more common causes are anemia, lack of protein, B-vitamin deficiency, hypothyroidism, female hormone imbalance, male pattern baldness, chemotherapy, autoimmunity, and numerous drugs. As you can see, many of the causes are nutrition related.

Poor nutrition may be due to a poor diet in which adequate protein, iron, vitamins, minerals, plant compounds, and healthy fats are lacking. It can also be due to poor absorption of nutrients along the gastrointestinal (GI) tract. The result is that the body does not obtain the nutrients necessary to produce or retain hair in the hair follicles, and scalp skin integrity is also compromised. Without proper nutrition, hair follicles may shrink and no longer support hair growth or retention.

Probiotics of many kinds improve nutrient absorption along the GI tract and support hair follicles and scalp skin. They do this in many ways, including:

- Preventing intestinal permeability so that your intestinal cells maintain their integrity, allow for proper nutrient absorption, and disallow absorption of molecules that are damaging to the body
- Providing an environment for digestive enzymes to work
- Breaking down antinutrients in foods so that micronutrients are freed from foods and absorbed
- Producing short-chain fatty acids to nourish intestinal cells
- Moving food along the GI tract at the appropriate pace
- Preventing an overabundance of pathogens that cause inflammation and stress in your intestine and scalp skin
- Supporting moisture balance and adequate blood flow in the scalp

Many topical hair-loss treatments promise to deliver a healthy-looking mane of hair, but include harsh chemicals that can compromise the health of your scalp and that may be absorbed internally, putting stress on your liver and other detoxification organs. Oral probiotics, along with a nutritious diet, are a nontoxic way to support hair growth and lessen hair loss.

88: COMBATS NAIL FUNGUS

Nail fungus can cause nails to bend, thicken, crumble, appear yellowish, and even separate from the nail bed. Toenails are a common location for this to happen, because they are often in dark, moist environments, but it can happen under fingernails too.

Several different types of fungi can cause nail fungus, entering the nail bed through injury to the nail or from fungus on the skin of the feet. This is why it is important to wear shoes suited to the type of activity, and to wear sandals around pools, locker rooms, and communal showers. It is also important to keep the skin on your feet moisturized enough to prevent cracks that are an entry point for fungus.

Another factor that plays a role in nail fungus is circulation. Impaired circulation limits the amount of nutrients and immune molecules that nourish nails and detect invaders like fungus, and it also limits the amount of cellular waste that is removed from nail beds. Type 2 diabetes, cardiovascular disease, immunocompromised states, and sedentary behavior increase your risk of acquiring nail fungus and decrease your ability to eliminate it.

Probiotics taken internally can help your nails get the nutrients they need from food for healthy growth. They can also increase moisture levels in your skin so that your skin is less likely to crack, and they improve circulation, waste removal, and immune function so that you are less likely to succumb to nail fungus, and may be better able to resolve it.

Probiotic products applied topically can battle nail fungus. One product, Cruex Nail Fungal Nail Revitalizing Gel, contains Bonicel, a patented fermentation product from a *Bacillus coagulans* probiotic bacterium, demonstrated to restore nail health. This product shows that fermentation products from probiotics can contribute to health even when live probiotics are absent.

89: MAKES NAILS STRONGER

Nails are a visible sign of personal care. Many women and men do not feel pulled together unless they have professionally done manicures and pedicures. A walk down the beauty aisle at your local store presents you with many options for brightly colored and muted nail polishes, nail buffers, nail strengtheners, and even artificial nails, all with the promise of providing you with strong, beautiful nails. The answer to healthy, strong, attractive nails does not lie in the beauty aisle, however.

Nails are also a visible sign of health. Dirty, jagged, thickened, and yellowed nails reflect an internal environment that differs from the environment that results in clean, filed, strong, white-edged nails. In order to have healthy nails, you have to have the right nutrients and the internal environment that supports the absorption of those nutrients and the elimination of wastes.

Nails are primarily composed of keratin, a strong protein. But in addition to adequate protein intake, you need minerals such as calcium, magnesium, and zinc, among others, and vitamins A, B, and C, at a minimum. You also need healthy nail beds, with adequate moisture, circulation, and waste removal.

Oral probiotics keep your gastrointestinal system intact so your body is able to digest foods you eat and absorb the nutrients from them that it needs for strong nails and healthy nail beds. They are capable of making some vitamins and supporting other microbiota that make others. Probiotics also affect your cardiovascular system and your thyroid hormones, thus affecting your circulation and your rate of nail growth. And they do all of this from the inside of your body! Instead of trying to have strong, beautiful nails by applying questionable products on the outside, nourish them from the inside with the benefits of probiotics.

90: BUILDS STRONGER BONES

Osteoporosis is a condition characterized by weak bones. Despite what you may have heard, both women and men are candidates for osteoporosis, especially with age. Broken hips are highly associated with disability and mortality risk.

Osteoporosis drug treatments usually aim to prevent bone breakdown, but strong bones are about more than just calcium and denseness. Your bone cells work to build new bone and remove older bone so that bone stays strong and flexible. Blocking the breakdown may result in denser bones, but those bones are not strong, nor flexible, and are prone to dying from lack of remodeling.

To have strong bones, you have to provide the correct building materials and supporting nutrients, such as protein, numerous minerals in addition to calcium, and vitamins. You also have to provide healthy levels of stress to bone, such as in weight-bearing exercise, so that the bone reacts to the stressor and becomes stronger.

Unlike drugs that only prevent bone breakdown, probiotics work at the level of helping you digest and absorb the nutrients needed for strong bones. They control levels of pathogenic microbes in the gut that produce inflammatory chemicals that can stimulate bone breakdown. Probiotics also help bone cells take in minerals needed for bone growth.

Probiotics cannot get you off the couch to do weight-bearing exercise, nor can they spoon-feed you the nutrients you need for bone health, but they perform many functions that serve to build and maintain strong, healthy bones.

TO MAKE A BONE-BUILDING PROTEIN SHAKE

This recipe combines bone-building nutrients with the power of live cultures.

8 ounces plain goat's, cow's, or
  alternative-milk kefir
½ cup frozen blueberries
1 large handful mixed salad greens
1 serving protein powder
1 teaspoon coconut oil or flax oil
Stevia to taste

Blend all the ingredients in a blender. Enjoy!

91: CALMS PSORIASIS

Raised red, itchy, and possibly painful silvery-scaly patches of dry skin that recur can be both uncomfortable and embarrassing. These are not ordinary dry skin patches, however, and may be a sign of a type of autoimmune psoriasis, a skin condition in which the body launches an inflammation attack against itself. Patches like these should be seen by a dermatologist or an immune specialist because in some cases they can be paired with psoriatic arthritis or other autoimmune diseases.

Psoriasis occurs when immature skin cells pile up on the surface of the skin due to activation of the immune system. Psoriasis is believed to have a genetic susceptibility that is activated by environmental factors such as a bacterial infection, antibiotic treatments, or other autoimmune diseases.

Typical treatments for psoriasis are topical creams based on steroids, vitamin D3, vitamin A derivatives, coal tar, or medications that slow the growth of skin cells; ultraviolet light therapy; or immune-suppressing oral drugs.

Since psoriasis is an immune-system-driven condition with known skin microbiome disruption, there is potential for probiotics to help. Probiotics are capable of reducing the microbiome disruption that leads to inflammation in the skin and overactivation of the immune system. They can also directly influence the immune system, tipping it back toward an anti-inflammatory state.

Several species of *Lactobacillus* and *Bifidobacterium* are known to be able to reduce the inflammatory molecules involved in psoriasis. While probiotics may or may not be able to replace conventional treatments in the future, they may help you now to reduce the uncomfortable and embarrassing signs of psoriasis.

92: MINIMIZES ROSACEA

Rosacea is a skin disorder, primarily on the face, characterized by facial redness with or without bumps or pimples, skin thickening, and eye irritation. It typically flares up and then goes into remission. What may begin as frequent blushing or flushing can progress to persistent redness with small, visible blood vessels and facial discomfort. In its severe form, disfigurement of the nose or face can result due to skin thickening.

Triggers of rosacea flare-ups differ from person to person, with various foods, beverages, emotional states, personal-care products, temperature, humidity changes, medical conditions, medications, and physical exertion noted as triggers. Sun exposure is the leading cause of flare-ups, so nontoxic sunscreen use is recommended daily. Skin-care products should be as gentle as possible, without harsh chemicals such as sodium laurel (laureth) sulfate and numerous parabens.

The exact cause of rosacea is unknown, but its symptoms are commonly treated with oral and topical treatments such as oral and topical antibiotics, laser therapy, and even surgery. Antibiotics kill bacteria. Interestingly, rosacea is known to be associated with gut dysbiosis, a disruption in balanced levels of microbes in the gastrointestinal (GI) tract, as well as skin microbiome dysbiosis. Treatment with antibiotics temporarily improves or resolves rosacea, but there may be a longer-lasting solution without the undesirable side effects of antibiotics: probiotics.

Probiotics excel at helping the body to correct dysbiosis, both in the GI tract as well as on the skin. Probiotics help improve skin moisture and elasticity, reduce redness, and reduce inflammation caused at the site of the rosacea as well as caused internally by pathogens in the GI tract. Probiotics also improve digestion of nutritious foods and absorption of nutrients necessary for healthy skin. Adding daily probiotics to your rosacea care program may lessen the symptoms and causes.

93: REDUCES DIAPER RASH

Diaper rash is common in infants and toddlers as well as in adults who wear disposable underwear. Urine and acidic stool break down the skin's natural barrier protection with the chronic wetness that is present in the warm environment of the diaper.

Many times diaper rash can be prevented or treated with a simple zinc oxide cream, but sometimes the rash can turn into a mild skin infection with a yeast such as *Candida albicans*. Usually the skin at the anus is infected first because *Candida* is a routine inhabitant of the digestive tract that is normally kept under control by beneficial bacteria and yeasts there. Once in the warm, moist environment of the diaper, though, it takes advantage of the opportunity to grow. From there, the infection spreads to the genitals, creases, thighs, and even abdomen if not dealt with early enough. The skin becomes red and irritated with large raised portions surrounded by small, infected, pimple-like lesions.

Typical treatment for a *Candida*-associated diaper infection is antifungal medication, given topically or orally. However, many fungi such as *Candida* are resistant or becoming resistant to the arsenal of antifungal medications.

Allergic reaction to antifungal medication is another concern. A better option is to control the population of *Candida* at its source in the digestive tract with nutritious food and probiotics.

Numerous probiotics have antagonist activity against *Candida* species. They are able to prevent it from attaching to intestinal tract tissues, prevent it from becoming invasive, control the population so that toxins released from *Candida* are minimized, and even kill it. Additionally, probiotics can keep skin hydrated and help to keep the skin and intestinal barrier intact.

Change diapers frequently, especially after soiling, and use probiotics daily to prevent infectious diaper rash from becoming an issue.

94: IMPROVES DRY SKIN

Dry skin is itchy and uncomfortable, especially when clothing or socks rub up against it. The real danger with dry skin, however, lies in the ability of the skin to crack, causing fissures that allow the outside world access to your inner tissues resulting in tender, inflamed skin and infections.

Genetics plays a role in skin dryness, as do heat and humidity conditions, but most dry skin is caused by excessive washing with products that strip the skin of its covering. Your skin naturally produces antimicrobial compounds and sebum, an oily substance, to moisturize, protect, and nourish the outer layers of skin. Although topically applied moisturizers may help with skin dryness temporarily, they have to be reapplied frequently. Many moisturizers contain ingredients that are toxic to your body, such as petrolatum (petroleum jelly), endocrine-hormone-disrupting parabens, antibacterials, synthetic hormones, synthetic fragrances, and preservatives.

The state of your gut health affects your skin, so oral probiotics should be a part of your natural skin-care routine. Probiotics taken internally help suppress water loss from the skin and improve plumpness of the skin to reduce dry skin. They regulate the immune system to suppress inflammatory chemicals from attacking the skin's collagen and structure. They also make skin-friendly nutrients more available and absorbable. Additionally, probiotics reduce pathogenic bacteria in your digestive tract that contribute to inflammation in your body, including your skin.

Applied topically, probiotics or their fermentation products provide protection to the skin to maintain a normal skin barrier. Probiotic fermentation products in a patented formula called *Bonicel* have shown efficacy in clinical trials for reducing dry skin.

You may be predisposed to some level of dry skin and/or live in an arid environment, but by avoiding harsh skin products and using probiotics you may be able to achieve the moisturized skin you have dreamed of.

95: SOOTHES SKIN REDNESS

A bit of redness on your cheeks makes you look like you have a healthy glow. You can naturally get that redness from being out in the cold or exercising, but what if redness is nearly always present, on your cheeks or elsewhere, and what if it is more irritated looking and feeling than healthy looking?

Persistent, uncomfortable redness on your skin is a sign that something is out of balance. It could be that you have contact dermatitis from clothing, bedding, personal-care products, or laundry products. It could be lack of sufficient circulation, particularly if the redness is on the legs. It could be eczema, psoriasis, rosacea, dryness, or an allergic reaction. If the redness is very itchy and seems to be spreading rapidly, seek medical help promptly because that could be a sign of cellulitis, an infection in the skin that can become serious quickly, or a fungal infection such as ringworm.

There are many reasons for persistent redness in your skin, but trying to treat it from the outside only is not addressing the internal reaction to whatever is causing it. The health of your gastrointestinal tract influences the health of your skin, and probiotics have a positive influence on both.

Numerous probiotics taken internally reduce the unnatural redness in your skin by contributing to maintenance of gut and skin integrity, assisting in digestion and absorption of skin-friendly nutrients, and controlling pathogens that contribute to inflammation in your skin and body. They also regulate your immune system to suppress inflammatory chemicals from attacking skin and blood vessels.

Having a healthy glow is different than having random redness in your skin. Have the redness diagnosed so you know what you are dealing with, and use probiotics and a nutritious diet and healthy lifestyle to help resolve it.

96: DIMINISHES WRINKLES

Wrinkles are an unwelcome sight for many people as they are obvious signs of aging. Antiwrinkle and antiaging creams and serums promise to restore the youth-like appearance of skin, but most of them are filled with questionable ingredients such as hormones or hormone derivatives, endocrine-disrupting parabens, petrochemicals, or harsh acids. Care must be taken with products applied to the skin because most ingredients are absorbed and can affect your entire body with a toxic burden. Hormone-like ingredients can disrupt your body's natural balance of hormones.

As skin ages, it loses collagen, which contributes to its plumpness and smoothness. It also loses the ability to hold onto moisture and maintain its barrier protection. Free radicals hold part of the blame for wrinkles by damaging collagen, which is why smoking and toxin exposure increases wrinkles. Free radicals are also produced by interactions with pathogenic bacteria in your gastrointestinal tract. Luckily, probiotics work to control and reduce those pathogens.

Probiotics taken internally also work to improve skin hydration, maintain plumpness of the skin, and improve skin elasticity, all of which reduce wrinkle depth. They accomplish this in various ways: regulating the immune system to suppress inflammatory chemicals from attacking the collagen and structure of the skin; protecting the liver so that it can neutralize toxins and excess hormones; and making skin-friendly nutrients more available to your body. Applied topically, probiotics and their fermentation products can provide antioxidant protection to the skin to help guard against free-radical damage, lessen fine lines and wrinkles, and maintain a normal skin barrier. Bonicel, a patented *Bacillus* fermentation product, has shown efficacy in decreasing wrinkles.

Nourishing skin from the inside reduces the effects of aging without the need for mystery ingredients. Aging is a normal part of life, but you can keep a more youthful appearance with probiotics!

97: WHITENS AND STRENGTHENS TEETH

The quest for pearly whites has many people bleaching, using abrasive cleaners and "whiteners," and using fluoride treatments on their teeth. Those treatments may achieve results, but success may come at the price of sensitive and eroded teeth, fluorosis, and potential health problems. The truth is, not everyone can have naturally dazzling, ultra-bright white teeth. Natural tooth color is largely determined by the color of dentine below the enamel and on the thickness and opaqueness of the enamel, and those begin to be determined in utero. Many variables can impact the outcome, such as genetics, levels of nutrients, injury, excessive fluoride, circulation, and hormone levels both in the womb and out.

If you must live with your baseline tooth color, what can you do to keep it as white as possible? Stains from things such as red wine, black tea, curry, and colored sodas can be on the enamel itself or on the plaque on the teeth. Reducing plaque by eating a nutritious diet including probiotics and foods and drinks with live cultures, along with proper hygiene, can reduce stained plaque and keep gums healthy. Foods and drinks with live cultures or probiotics may reduce stains on enamel.

Another way to keep your teeth as white as possible is to keep them strong. Probiotics improve digestion of foods and absorption of nutrients necessary for strong teeth from the inside. They also promote remineralization of teeth by minerals in saliva on the outside.

Dazzling white teeth are desirable for many people, but treatments to achieve them could ultimately be detrimental to your teeth and your health. Eating a nutritious diet, engaging in routine dental hygiene, avoiding tooth-degrading sodas, and enjoying sources of probiotics and live cultures can help you have healthy pearly whites.

98: BATTLES THRUSH

Thrush is an infection of the mouth and oral cavity with the yeast *Candida*. The most obvious symptom is a white film or cottage-cheese-like substance coating the tongue and surfaces of the oral cavity, but thrush can cause discomfort or pain, particularly when a person tries to chew. Thrush can occur in people of all ages, from babies to the elderly, especially when the immune system is compromised. Breastfeeding babies may transfer *Candida* to the mothers' nipples. The most commonly occurring form of *Candida* in thrush is *albicans*.

Candida albicans normally inhabits the mouth and the rest of the gastrointestinal (GI) tract and is kept under control by beneficial bacteria and yeasts there. Once given the opportunity to grow, however, such as with antibiotic use, oral immune-suppression drug use, lack of proper nutrition, smoking, antibacterial mouthwashes, or use of topical or inhaled corticosteroids, it easily expands its infective capabilities. It can spread to the pharynx and esophagus, become invasive, and be hard to eliminate. In severe cases, *Candida* infections can spread to the bloodstream and become life-threatening.

Typical treatment for thrush is antifungal medication, given topically or orally. However, many fungi such as *Candida* are resistant or becoming resistant to many over-the-counter and prescription-only antifungal medications. Allergic reaction to antifungal medications is another concern. A better option is to use nutritious food and probiotics to control the population of *Candida* at its source in the GI tract.

Probiotics in general can battle *Candida* species. They are able to prevent it from attaching to intestinal tract tissues, prevent it from becoming virulent and invasive, control the population so that released toxins are minimized, and even eliminate it. Additionally, probiotics can keep skin hydrated and help keep the skin barrier inside the oral cavity intact so that thrush resolves.

99: AIDS IN WEIGHT GAIN

It may seem like nearly everyone is trying to lose weight, but there are people who are trying to gain it. Sometimes the inability to gain weight is insufficient calorie intake or distorted proportions of fats, proteins, and carbohydrates. This may not be recognized until you document your food intake. Insufficient intake may be due to medications or excessive stimulants, which decrease appetite, to health situations such as hospitalization, dementia, or eating disorders, or to ignoring hunger pangs while under stress.

In many cases, gut dysfunction is to blame. Autoimmune gastrointestinal (GI) disorders such as celiac disease and Crohn's disease cause inflammation and destruction in the part of the GI tract, the small intestine, in which most of digestion and nutrient absorption takes place. Without proper digestion and absorption, nutrients are eliminated and weight gain is hampered.

It does not take a diagnosable autoimmune disease to affect gut dysfunction. GI dysbiosis, an imbalance in gut microbiota weighted toward pathogens and opportunists, is a common cause of an inability to gain weight for the same reasons as the diseases. Small intestinal bacterial overgrowth (SIBO) leads to inflammation, with digestive enzyme activity and nutrient absorption hindered. SIBO can also cause brain fog or emotional and mood symptoms resulting in lack of interest in preparing nutritious foods. This leads to a vicious circle of not enough nutrients and not enough nutrient absorption.

Fortunately, probiotics can be effective in repairing intestinal permeability found in the small intestine autoimmunity diseases and SIBO. They restore microbial balance and reduce inflammation and damaging oxidative stress. If you find it hard to gain weight, make sure you are taking in enough nutrients and using probiotics and probiotic-friendly food to restore your microbiome to a more balanced state.

100: HELPS WITH WEIGHT LOSS

You dread stepping on the scale and avoid looking at your profile in the mirror because you know you gained weight and need to lose some. You tried every diet on the market to no avail. Your frustration level is high, but you do not need to give up hope. The first thing to do is to love yourself regardless of your weight so that your emotions and stress levels do not sabotage your efforts. You can love yourself while working toward self-improvement.

There are many things that may be contributing to your inability to lose weight. Insulin resistance is a big one. Medication use is another. Subclinical thyroid problems, sex hormone imbalances, mindless eating, excess stress, insufficient muscle mass, age, genetics, lack of sleep, lack of exercise...the list goes on and on.

One thing that is often overlooked is gut health. Gut microbiota can affect food intake choices, appetite, and body weight and composition. Dysbiosis, an imbalance in the gut microbiota with a shift favoring pathogens and opportunists, is common in overweight people. The pathogens and opportunists create an inflammatory situation that affects insulin and other hormones, resulting in the inability to lose weight.

Numerous *Lactobacillus* and *Bifidobacterium* probiotics have the ability to affect blood glucose levels, insulin resistance, thyroid and sex hormone levels, and other metabolic markers involved in weight loss, and control the pathogens and opportunists contributing to inflammation.

A diet high in vegetables, fruit, and fiber, and probiotic intake, supports a more diverse gut microbiome, which in turn helps weight loss. Instead of waiting for the next magical diet or weight-loss supplement to arrive, focus on improving your gut health with probiotics and foods and drinks with live cultures, in addition to maintaining healthy lifestyle factors.

REFERENCES

Probiotics and Their Many Health Benefits

P.A. Mackowiak. "Recycling Metchnikoff: Probiotics, the Intestinal Microbiome and the Quest for Long Life," *Frontiers in Public Health* 1.52 (2013).

J.A. Panyko. *Probiotics: How to Use Them to Your Advantage*. Denver, Colorado. Outskirts Press. Print.

Soothes Achy Joints

"Osteoarthritis," *Arthritis Research UK*, www.arthritisresearchuk.org/arthritis-information/conditions/osteoarthritis.aspx (accessed January 26, 2017).

Lowers Rheumatoid Arthritis Activity

L. Xiaofei et al. "*Lactobacillus salivarius* Isolated from Patients with Rheumatoid Arthritis Suppresses Collagen-Induced Arthritis and Increases Treg Frequency in Mice," *Journal of Interferon & Cytokine Research* 36.12 (2016).

B. Zamani et al. "Clinical and metabolic response to probiotic supplementation in patients with rheumatoid arthritis: a randomized, double-blind, placebo-controlled trial," *International Journal of Rheumatic Diseases* 19.9 (2016): 869–879.

Improves Asthma

J. Liu et al. "Probiotics enhance the effect of allergy immunotherapy on regulating antigen specific B cell activity in asthma patients," *American Journal of Translational Research* 8.12 (2016): 5256–5270.

M.A. van de Pol et al. "Synbiotics reduce allergen-induced T-helper 2 response and improve peak expiratory flow in allergic asthmatics," *Allergy* 66.1 (2011): 39–47.

Shows Promise for Helping Autism

Ohio State University. "Autism symptoms improve after fecal transplant, small study finds: Parents report fewer behavioral and gastrointestinal problems; gut microbiome changes," *ScienceDaily*, ScienceDaily, January 23, 2017, www.sciencedaily.com/releases/2017/01/170123094638.html (accessed January 24, 2017).

Reduces Vaginal Inflammation

J.A. Panyko. "Aerobic Vaginitis—Similar To, But Different From, BV," *Power of Probiotics*, PowerofProbiotics.com, www.powerofprobiotics.com/Aerobic-vaginitis.html (accessed January 26, 2017).

Combats Bacterial Vaginosis

J.A. Panyko. "Treatment of Bacterial Vaginosis with Probiotics," *Power of Probiotics*, PowerofProbiotics.com, www.powerofprobiotics.com/Treatment-of-bacterial-vaginosis-with-probiotics.html (accessed January 26, 2017).

Reduces Risks Associated with Burn Injury

A. Argenta et al. "Local Application of Probiotic Bacteria Prophylaxes against Sepsis and Death Resulting from Burn Wound Infection," *PLoS ONE* 11.10 (2016): 1–16.

A. Makhdoom et al. "Role of Probiotics in the Management of Burns Patients," *World Journal of Medical Sciences* 11.3 (2014): 417–421.

Offers Help in Liver Cancer Prevention

J. Li et al. "Probiotics modulated gut microbiota suppresses hepatocellular carcinoma growth in mice," *Proceedings of the National Academy of Sciences of the United States of America* 113.9 (2016): E1306–E1315.

Reduces Cardiovascular Disease Risks

"Cardiovascular Diseases," *World Health Organization*, World Health Organization, www.who.int/topics/cardiovascular_diseases/en (accessed January 31, 2017).

Helps to Balance Cholesterol

J.A. Panyko. "*Lactobacillus reuteri* NCIMB 30242 Is a Cholesterol-Reducing Probiotic," *Power of Probiotics*, PowerofProbiotics.com, www.powerofprobiotics.com/Lactobacillus-reuteri-NCIMB-30242.html (accessed January 20, 2017).

May Reduce Duration and Severity of Colds

"Common Cold," *Centers for Disease Control and Prevention*, US Department of Health & Human Services, www.cdc.gov/dotw/common-cold/index.html (accessed January 20, 2017).

Soothes Colic

C. de Weerth et al. "Crying in Infants," *Gut Microbes* 4.5 (2013): 416–421.

Relieves Constipation

J.A. Panyko. "Constipation: A Mostly-Preventable Regularity Problem," *Power of Probiotics*, PowerofProbiotics.com, www.powerofprobiotics.com/Constipation.html (accessed January 26, 2017).

Helps with Complications of Cystic Fibrosis

J.L. Anderson et al. "Effect of probiotics on respiratory, gastrointestinal and nutritional outcomes in patients with cystic fibrosis: A systematic review," *Journal of Cystic Fibrosis* 16.2 (2017): 186-197, epublished September 29, 2016 (accessed January 30, 2016).

Offers Help for Diabetes

"2014 National Diabetes Statistics Report," *Centers for Disease Control and Prevention*, US Department of Health & Human Services, www.cdc.gov/diabetes/data/statistics/2014statisticsreport.html (accessed January 30, 2017).

"Diabetes," *World Health Organization*, World Health Organization, www.who.int/mediacentre/factsheets/fs312/en (accessed January 30, 2017).

Lessens Risk of Gallstones

"Gallstones," *Mayo Clinic*, Mayo Foundation for Medical Education and Research, www.mayoclinic.org/diseases-conditions/gallstones/home/ovc-20231394 (accessed February 2, 2017).

May Reduce Postsurgical Infections

"Surgical Site Infection (SSI) Event," *Procedure-Associated Module, SSI, Centers for Disease Control and Prevention*, US Department of Health & Human Services, January 2017. Print.

Enhances Female Fertility

"Female infertility," *Mayo Clinic*, Mayo Foundation for Medical Education and Research, www.mayoclinic.org/diseases-conditions/female-infertility/symptoms-causes/dxc-20214762 (accessed January 29, 2017).

Enhances Male Fertility

M.A. Ghoneim and S.S. Moselhy. "Antioxidant status and hormonal profile reflected by experimental feeding of probiotics," *Toxicology and Industrial Health* 32.4 (2016): 741–750.

"Male infertility," *Mayo Clinic*, Mayo Foundation for Medical Education and Research, www.mayoclinic.org/diseases-conditions/male-infertility/basics/definition/con-20033113 (accessed January 29, 2017).

Reduces Kidney Burden

J.A. Panyko. "Chronic Kidney Disease (CKD): Probiotics Are a Missing Key," *Power of Probiotics,* PowerofProbiotics.com, www.powerofprobiotics.com/Chronic-kidney-disease.html (accessed February 2, 2017).

J.A. Panyko. "Renadyl: The Probiotic Supplement for Chronic Kidney Disease (CKD)," *Power of Probiotics,* PowerofProbiotics.com, www.powerofprobiotics.com/Renadyl.html (accessed February 2, 2017).

Lessens Risk of Kidney Stones

M. Liebman and I.A. Al-Wahsh. "Probiotics and Other Key Determinants of Dietary Oxalate Absorption," *Advances in Nutrition* 2 (2011): 254–260.

C.D. Scales et al. "Prevalence of kidney stones in the United States," *European Urology* 62.1 (2012): 160–165.

May Reduce Risk of NAFLD

J.A. Panyko. "NAFLD: Can Liver Fat Be Helped by Probiotics?" *Power of Probiotics*, PowerofProbiotics.com, www.powerofprobiotics.com/NAFLD.html (accessed February 2, 2017).

May Help Prevent Conditions Leading to Lymphoma

"Lymphoma: Causes, Symptoms and Research," *MNT*, Medical News Today, www.medicalnewstoday.com/articles/146136.php (accessed February 2, 2017).

J.A. Panyko. "Probiotics and Lymphoma Prevention: Is There a Connection?" *Power of Probiotics*, PowerofProbiotics.com, www.powerofprobiotics.com/Lymphoma-prevention .html (accessed February 2, 2017).

Promotes Eye Health

L. Ma et al. "Lutein, Zeaxanthin and Meso-zeaxanthin Supplementation Associated with Macular Pigment Optical Density," *Nutrients* 8.7 (2016): 426.

Decreases Vaginal Dryness

J. Shen et al. "Effects of Low Dose Estrogen Therapy on the Vaginal Microbiomes of Women with Atrophic Vaginitis," *Scientific Reports* 6.24380 (2016).

Offers Help for MS Symptoms

"What Is MS?" *National Multiple Sclerosis Society*, National Multiple Sclerosis Society, www.nationalmssociety.org/What-is-MS (accessed February 3, 2017).

Lessens NEC Risk

J.A. Panyko. "Necrotizing Enterocolitis: Probiotics Can Help," *Power of Probiotics*, PowerofProbiotics.com, www.powerofprobiotics.com/Necrotizing-enterocolitis.html (accessed February 3, 2017).

S.C. Sawh et al. "Prevention of necrotizing enterocolitis with probiotics: a systematic review and meta-analysis," *PeerJ* 4 (2016): e2429.

Helps Reduce Risk of Acute Pancreatitis

F. Lutgendorff et al. "Probiotics enhance pancreatic glutathione biosynthesis and reduce oxidative stress in experimental acute pancreatitis," *American Journal of Physiology: Gastrointestinal and Liver Physiology* 295.5 (2008): G1111–G1121.

"What Is Pancreatitis?" *WebMD*, WebMD, LLC, www.webmd.com/digestive-disorders/digestive-diseases-pancreatitis#2 (accessed February 3, 2017).

Battles Periodontal Disease

"Periodontal (Gum) Disease: Causes, Symptoms, and Treatments," *National Institute of Dental and Craniofacial Research*, National Institutes of Health, www.nidcr.nih.gov/OralHealth/Topics/GumDiseases/PeriodontalGumDisease.htm (accessed February 3, 2017).

S. Xu et al. "The Association between Periodontal Disease and the Risk of Myocardial Infarction: A Pooled Analysis of Observational Studies," *BMC Cardiovascular Disorders* 17.1 (2017): 50.

Eases PMS

A.R. Kroll-Desrosiers et al. "Recreational Physical Activity and Premenstrual Syndrome in Young Adult Women: A Cross-Sectional Study," *PLoS ONE* 12.1 (2017): e0169728.

Impedes Pneumonia Pathogens

L. Khailova et al. "*Lactobacillus rhamnosus* GG treatment improves intestinal permeability and modulates inflammatory response and homeostasis of spleen and colon in experimental model of *Pseudomonas aeruginosa* pneumonia," *Clinical Nutrition*, epublished October 1, 2016, www.ncbi.nlm.nih.gov/pubmed/27745813 (accessed February 4, 2017).

"Pneumonia," *Mayo Clinic*, Mayo Foundation for Medical Education and Research, www.mayoclinic.org/diseases-conditions/pneumonia/home/ovc-20204676 (accessed February 4, 2014).

Fights Pouchitis

"Pouchitis," *Cleveland Clinic*, Cleveland Clinic, http://my.clevelandclinic.org/health/articles/pouchitis (accessed February 4, 2016).

Reduces Risk of Preterm Birth

A.B. Dunn et al. "The Microbiome and Complement Activation: A Mechanistic Model for Preterm Birth," *Biological Research for Nursing* 19.3 (2017): 295-307, epublished January 11, 2017, http://journals.sagepub.com/doi/abs/10.1177/1099800416687648 (accessed January 14, 2017).

"Preterm Birth," *Centers for Disease Control and Prevention*, US Department of Health & Human Services, www.cdc.gov/reproductivehealth/maternalinfanthealth/pretermbirth.htm (accessed February 5, 2017).

Addresses Radiation Enteritis

"Radiation enteritis," *Canadian Cancer Society*, Canadian Cancer Society, www.cancer.ca/en/cancer-information/diagnosis-and-treatment/radiation-therapy/side-effects-of-radiation-therapy/radiation-to-the-abdomen/radiation-enteritis/?region=sk (accessed February 5, 2017).

J.P. Weiner et al. "Endoscopic and Non-endoscopic Approaches for the Management of Radiation-induced Rectal Bleeding," *World Journal of Gastroenterology* 22.31 (2016): 6972–6986.

Lessens Rotavirus Impact

G.A. Preidis et al. "Host Response to Probiotics Determined by Nutritional Status of Rotavirus-infected Neonatal Mice," *Journal of Pediatric Gastroenterology and Nutrition* 55.3 (2012): 299–307.

"Rotavirus," *Centers for Disease Control and Prevention*, US Department of Health & Human Services, www.cdc.gov/rotavirus/about/symptoms.html (accessed February 6, 2017).

Improves Short-Bowel Syndrome

Y. Kanamori et al. "Combination Therapy with *Bifidobacterium breve, Lactobacillus casei*, and Galactooligosaccharides Dramatically Improved the Intestinal Function in a Girl with Short Bowel Syndrome," *Digestive Diseases and Sciences* 46.9 (2001): 2010–2016.

"Short Bowel Syndrome," *National Institute of Diabetes and Digestive and Kidney Diseases*, National Institutes of Health, www.niddk.nih.gov/health-information/digestive-diseases/short-bowel-syndrome (accessed February 6, 2017).

Promotes Sinus Health

M. Hoggard et al. "Evidence of microbiota dysbiosis in chronic rhinosinusitis," *International Forum of Allergy & Rhinology* 7.3 (2017): 230-239, epublished November 23, 2016, www.ncbi.nlm.nih.gov/pubmed/27879060 (accessed February 16, 2017).

J.S. Schwartz et al. "Topical Probiotics as a Therapeutic Alternative for Chronic Rhinosinusitis: A Preclinical Proof of Concept," *American Journal of Rhinology & Allergy* 30.6 (2016): 202–205.

Enhances Sports Performance

A. Clark and N. Mach. "Exercise-induced stress behavior, gut-microbiota-brain axis and diet: a systematic review for athletes," *Journal of the International Society of Sports Nutrition* 13.43 (2016).

Limits Stomach Flu

"Viral gastroenteritis (stomach flu)," *Mayo Clinic*, Mayo Foundation for Medical Education and Research, www.mayoclinic.org/diseases-conditions/viral-gastroenteritis/basics/

definition/con-20019350 (accessed February 15, 2017).

Thwarts Stomach Ulcers

A.H. Cekin et al. "Use of Probiotics as an Adjuvant to Sequential *H. pylori* Eradication Therapy: Impact on Eradication Rates, Treatment Resistance, Treatment-Related Side Effects, and Patient Compliance," *Turkish Journal of Gastroenterology* 28.1 (2017): 3–11.

"Peptic ulcer," *Mayo Clinic*, Mayo Foundation for Medical Education and Research, www.mayoclinic.org/diseases-conditions/peptic-ulcer/home/ovc-20231363 (accessed February 17, 2017).

Lessens Toxic Shock Syndrome Risk

R.A. MacPhee et al. "Influence of the Vaginal Microbiota on Toxic Shock Syndrome Toxin 1 Production by *Staphylococcus aureus*," *Applied and Environmental Microbiology* 79.6 (2013): 1835–842.

Helps Consequences of Major Physical Trauma

C.E.M. Brathwaite et al. "Bacterial translocation occurs in humans after traumatic injury: Evidence using immunofluorescence," *Journal of Trauma and Acute Care Surgery* 34.4 (1993): 586–590.

Promotes Urinary Health

L. Brubaker and A.J. Wolfe. "The female urinary microbiota, urinary health and common urinary disorders," *Annals of Translational Medicine* 5.2 (2017).

Improves Alzheimer's Disease

E. Akbari et al. "Effect of Probiotic Supplementation on Cognitive Function and Metabolic Status in Alzheimer's Disease: A Randomized, Double-Blind and Controlled Trial," *Frontiers in Aging Neuroscience* 8.256 (2016).

Reduces Causes of Anxiety

M. Lyte. "Microbial Endocrinology in the Microbiome-Gut-Brain Axis: How Bacterial Production and Utilization of Neurochemicals Influence Behavior," *PLoS Pathogens* 9.11 (2013): e1003726.

May Help with Bipolar Disease

"Bipolar Disorder," *National Institute of Mental Health*, National Institutes of Health, www.nimh.nih.gov/health/topics/bipolar-disorder/index.shtml#part_145402 (accessed February 17, 2017).

A.A. Chrobak et al. "Interactions between the gut microbiome and the central nervous system and their role in schizophrenia, bipolar disorder and depression," *Archives of Psychiatry and Psychotherapy* 2 (2016): 5-11.

Alleviates Depression

J.A. Panyko. "Can Probiotics (Psychobiotics) Help with Depression?" *Power of Probiotics*, PowerofProbiotics.com, www.powerofprobiotics.com/Depression.html (accessed February 9, 2017).

Addresses Headaches

"Headache," *MedicineNet*, MedicineNet, Inc., www.medicinenet.com/headache/page2.htm (accessed February 9, 2017).

X. Wei et al. "Dural fibroblasts play a potential role in headache pathophysiology," *Pain* 155.7 (2014): 1238–1244.

Improves Hepatic Encephalopathy

J. Cordoba. "Hepatic Encephalopathy: From the Pathogenesis to the New Treatments," *International Scholarly Research Notices*, article ID 236268 (2014).

L.N. Zhao et al. "Probiotics Can Improve the Clinical Outcomes of Hepatic Encephalopathy: An Update Meta-Analysis," *Clinics and Research in Hepatology and Gastroenterology* 39.6 (2015): 674–682.

May Help Schizophrenia

"Schizophrenia," *National Institute of Mental Health*, National Institutes of Health, www.nimh.nih.gov/health/topics/schizophrenia/index.shtml (accessed February 18, 2017).

H. Karakula-Juchnowicz et al. "The Brain-Gut Axis Dysfunctions and Hypersensitivity to Food Antigens in the Etiopathogenesis of Schizophrenia," *Psychiatria Polska* 50.4 (2016): 747-760.

Minimizes Acne

J.A. Panyko. "Acne Is More Than a Few Breakouts," *Power of Probiotics*, PowerofProbiotics.com, www.powerofprobiotics.com/Acne.html (accessed February 19, 2017).

Fights Athlete's Foot

"Athlete's Foot," *eMedicineHealth*, WebMD, LLC, www.emedicinehealth.com/athletes_foot-health/article_em.htm#Topic%20Overview (accessed February 19, 2017).

Battles Bad Breath

H.J. Jang et al. "Comparative Study on the Characteristics of *Weissella cibaria* CMU and Probiotic Strains for Oral Care," *Molecules* 21.12 (2016): E1752.

Lessens Sweaty Body Odor

C. Callewaert et al. "Characterization of *Staphylococcus* and *Corynebacterium* Clusters in the Human Axillary Region," *PLoS ONE* 8.8 (2013): e70538.

Improves Fishy Body Odor

J.A. Panyko. "TMAU (Trimethylaminuria): The Causes, Types and Triggers," *Power of Probiotics*, PowerofProbiotics.com, www.powerofprobiotics.com/TMAU.html (accessed February 20, 2017).

Relieves Eczema

H. Zheng et al. "Altered Gut Microbiota Composition Associated with Eczema in Infants," *PLoS ONE* 11.11 (2016): e0166026.

Calms Psoriasis

"Questions and Answers about Psoriasis," *National Institute of Arthritis and Musculoskeletal and Skin Diseases*, National Institutes of Health, www.niams.nih.gov/health_info/psoriasis (accessed February 22, 2017).

Z. Zákostelská et al. "Intestinal Microbiota Promotes Psoriasis-Like Skin Inflammation by Enhancing Th17 Response," *PLoS ONE* 11.7 (2016): e0159539.

Minimizes Rosacea

"Factors That May Trigger Rosacea Flare-Ups," *National Rosacea Society*, National Rosacea Society, www.rosacea.org/patients/materials/triggers.php (accessed February 23, 2017).

Reduces Diaper Rash

J. Mohamadi et al. "Anti-fungal resistance in candida isolated from oral and diaper rash candidiasis in neonates," *Bioinformation* 10.11 (2014): 667–670.

Battles Thrush

J. Mohamadi et al. "Anti-fungal resistance in candida isolated from oral and diaper rash candidiasis in neonates," *Bioinformation* 10.11 (2014): 667–670.

INDEX

A

B

F

J

Joints, achy, soothing, 21

K

Kidneys, reducing burden of, CKD and, 51

Kidney stones, lessening risk of, 51

L

Lactobacillus probiotics
  about: overview of, 17
  acne and, 89
  acute pancreatitis (AP) and, 61
  Alzheimer's disease (AD) and, 79
  anemia and, 20
  anxiety and, 80
  bacterial vaginosis (BV) and, 26
  bad breath and, 92
  bodily locations of, 17
  body odor and, 95
  brain fog and, 82
  burn injury risks and, 27
  cholesterol balance and, 32
  colic and, 34
  depression and, 83
  heartburn and, 43
  hepatic encephalopathy (HE) and, 85
  irritability and, 86
  kidney function, kidney stones and, 51, 52
  lactose intolerance and, 53
  male fertility and, 49
  necrotizing enterocolitis (NEC) risk and, 60
  periodontal disease (PD) and, 62, 65
  psoriasis and, 108
  reducing aging from sun exposure, 90

  rheumatoid arthritis (RA) and, 22
  rotavirus impact and, 68
  seasonal allergies and, 19
  short-bowel syndrome (SBS) and, 69
  sources of, 17
  stomach ulcers and, 73
  toxic shock syndrome (TSS) and, 75
  urinary health and, 77
  vaginal dryness and, 58
  vaginal inflammation and, 25
  weight loss and, 117

Lactococcus probiotics, 17, 20, 61

Lactose intolerance, improving, 53

Leuconostoc probiotics, 17

Liver
  cancer prevention, 30
  hepatic encephalopathy (HE) and, 85
  protecting function of, 54
  reducing risk of NAFLD, 55
  whitening eyes and, 101

Lymphoma, 56

M

Macular degeneration (MD), 57

Major trauma (MT), 76

MD (macular degeneration), 57

Metchnikoff, Élie, 14

Microbes
  about: overview of benefits, 13–14, 15–16
  bodily locations of, 14–15
  importance to health, 14
  killing pathogens, 15
  microbiome and, 13
  in skin, 14–15
  types of probiotic, 16–17. *See also specific types of microbes*

MS (multiple sclerosis), helping symptoms, 59

Mucus
  bad breath, microbes and, 92
  cystic fibrosis (CF) and, 36
  microbes in, 15
  radiation enteritis (RE) and, 67
  sinus health, microbes, 70
Multiple sclerosis (MS), helping symptoms, 59
Musculoskeletal structure
  osteoarthritis (OA) and probiotics, 21
  rheumatoid arthritis (RA) and, 22
  soothing achy joints, 21

N

NAFLD (nonalcoholic fatty liver disease), 55
Nail(s)
  fungus, 105
  making stronger, 106
Necrotizing enterocolitis (NEC), lessening, 60
Nonalcoholic fatty liver disease (NAFLD), 55

O

Oral health
  battling thrush, 115
  bleeding gums and, 103
  fighting cavities and, 97
  periodontal disease (PD) and, 62
  whitening and strengthening teeth, 114
Osteoarthritis (OA) and probiotics, 21
Osteoporosis, fighting, 107

P

PB (preterm birth), reducing risk of, 66
Peptic ulcers, thwarting, 73
Periodontal disease (PD), battling, 62
PMS (premenstrual syndrome), easing, 63

Pneumonia pathogens, impeding, 64
Postsurgical infections, reducing, 47
Pouchitis, fighting, 65
Precautions and side effects, 16
Premenstrual syndrome (PMS), easing, 63
Preterm birth (PB), reducing risk of, 66
Probiotics
  about: overview of, 11–12
  as beneficial microbes, 11, 13
  cautions, 16
  concept origin, 14
  defined, 11, 13
  historical perspective, 13–14
  side effects, 16
  sources of, 14
  special benefits of, 14–16
  super potent forms, 13
  yogurt cultures and, 14
Psoriasis, calming, 108
Psychological issues
  anxiety and, 80
  bipolar disease (BD) and, 81
  brain fog, 82
  depression, 83
  irritability and, 86
  schizophrenia, 87

R

Radiation enteritis (RE), 67
Rash, diaper, 110
Redness, skin, 112
Rheumatoid arthritis (RA), 22
Rosacea, minimizing, 109
Rotavirus, lessening impact of, 68

S

Saccharomyces probiotics
  about: overview of, 17

bipolar disease (BD) and, 81
schizophrenia and, 87
sources of, 17
species of, 17
stomach ulcers and, 73
yeast infections and, 78
SBS (short-bowel syndrome), improving, 69
Schizophrenia, helping, 87
Seasonal allergy reactions, lessening, 19
Short-bowel syndrome (SBS), improving, 69
SIBO (small intestinal bacterial overgrowth), 116
Side effects of probiotics, 16
Sinus health, promoting, 70
Skin
acne and, 89
cancer, 90
diminishing wrinkles, 113
dry, improving, 111
microbes in, 14–15
psoriasis and, 108
redness, soothing, 112
reducing aging from sun exposure, 90
relieving eczema, 100
rosacea and, 109
Small intestinal bacterial overgrowth (SIBO), 69, 116
Smelly gas, reducing, 102
Sources of probiotics, 14
Sports performance, enhancing, 71
Stomach flu, limiting, 72
Stomach ulcers, thwarting, 73
Streptococcus probiotics
about: overview of, 17
anemia and, 20
burn injury risks and, 27
cavities and, 97
colic and, 34

kidney function, kidney stones and, 51, 52
lactose intolerance and, 53
pneumonia and, 64
pouchitis and, 65
sources of, 17
species of, 17
Sugar cravings, reducing, 88
Sun exposure, reducing aging from, 90
Surgery, reducing infections after, 47
Sweaty body odor, lessening, 95

T

Teeth, fighting cavities in, 97
Thrush, battling, 115
Thyroid problems, 74
TMAU (trimethylaminuria), improving, 96
Toxic shock syndrome (TSS), 75
Trauma, major, 76
Trimethylaminuria (TMAU), improving, 96

U

Ulcers, stomach, thwarting, 73
Urinary tract, microbes in, 14
Urinary tract infection (UTI), 77

V

Vagina
aerobic vaginitis (AV) and, 25
bacterial vaginosis (BV) and, 26
dryness of, decreasing, 58
inflammation, 25
preterm birth risk and, 66
toxic shock syndrome (TSS) and, 75
urinary health and, 77

ABOUT THE AUTHOR

Jo A. Panyko, BS, MNT, is the author of several books and guides on the use of probiotics, including *Probiotics: How to Use Them to Your Advantage*. She is passionate about gut health and the influences of the gut microbiome and probiotics on health. Jo created the popular science-based website, PowerofProbiotics.com, to teach consumers and healthcare professionals about the importance of gastrointestinal health and probiotics.

Jo is a functional nutritionist in private practice, a nutrition consultant, and speaker; she holds a degree in engineering, is a professional member of the National Association of Nutrition Professionals, and is a volunteer nutrition educator.

In addition to her passion for investigating the links between diet, lifestyle, environment, and health, Jo enjoys precious time with her husband, children, dog, and friends. She gardens year-round, indoors and outside, to keep her sanity, and is often seen training for hiking and backpacking adventures.

You can visit her website for additional information to complement her books, sign up for her newsletter, and connect with her at PowerofProbiotics .com. You can also reach her on *Facebook* at Power of Probiotics and on *Twitter* @PowerOfProbiotx.